Gestational diabetes journal

Keeping your baby healthy

Book 2 of the Baby Steps to Gestational diabetes series

Created by Mathea Ford, RD/LD

Purpose and Introduction

What I have found through the emails and requests of my readers is that it is difficult to find information about a gestational diabetes diet that is actionable. I want you to know that is what I intend to provide in all my books and guides. You can take this guide and create a healthy meal plan, write it out, and track what you are doing so that you can improve your gestational diabetes condition.

I wrote this module with you in mind: the mom with gestational diabetes who does not know where to start or can't seem to get the answers that you need from other sources. This journal will provide information that is applicable to your gestational diabetes diet.

Who am I? I am a registered dietitian in the USA who has been working with patients for my entire 15 + years of experience. I had gestational diabetes just like you, for both of my pregnancies and I understand where you are and how it feels! Find all my books on Amazon on my author page: http://www.amazon.com/Mathea-Ford/e/B008E1E7IS/

My goals are simple – to give some answers and to create an understanding of what is typical. In this book, I will take you through the gestational diabetes diet and how your pregnancy progresses with the general information provided. It will not necessarily be what happens in your case, as everyone is an individual. I may simplify things in an effort to write them so that I feel you can learn the most from the information. This may mean that I don't say the exact things that your doctor would say. If you don't understand, please ask your doctor.

I want you to know, I am not a medical doctor and I am not aware of your particular condition. Information in this module is current as of publication, but may or may not have changed. This module is not meant to substitute for medical treatment for you, your friends, your caregivers, or your family members. You should not base treatment decisions solely on what is contained in this module. Develop your treatment plan with your doctors, nurses and the other medical professionals on your team. I recommend that you double-check any information with your medical team to verify if it applies to you.

In other words, I am not responsible for your medical care. I am providing this module for information and entertainment purposes, not medical diagnoses. Please consult with your doctor about any questions that you have about your particular case.

Gestational Diabetes Meal Plan Basics

This book is designed as a tool to aid you in keeping you and your baby as healthy as you can. You can track, document, and discuss your gestational diabetes so you can find out what is causing you problems and what you think is really working. You should take this book with you when you leave home and continue to write down your information, and make sure you take it to all your doctor's appointments. You can find out trends and issues by tracking your meals and blood sugars. I want you to have the best pregnancy you possibly can.

Gestational diabetes happens during pregnancy and you usually find out that you have it during weeks 24—28 of your pregnancy. You might have had gestational diabetes with one of your pregnancies before. Or you could be experiencing this for the first time! Either way—I know you are trying very hard to watch your meals and snacks and to keep your blood sugar under control.

I want to go over some quick information about gestational diabetes, but if you need a gestational diabetes cookbook or meal plans, I have another book. It's a gestational diabetes diet meal planning guide—you can find it at Amazon :

http://www.gestationaldiabetesdietmealplan.com/go/mealplanbook

In general, gestational diabetes happens during pregnancy and is "cured" when you deliver. It's caused by hormonal changes in your body, and it increases your blood sugar. The increased blood sugar can cause problems for you and your baby. It's best for moms to try to control the levels of blood sugars.

You can get a quick guide to all things related to gestational diabetes FOR FREE by signing up on our website for the mailing list where we provide lots of helpful information. Just go to our website at:

http://www.gestationaldiabetesdietmealplan.com

On the upper right side of the home page is the sign up. Once you have signed up, our book talks about blood sugar levels, exercise and using medications to control your blood sugars.

Basic Tips For Managing Gestational Diabetes

1. Watch your carbohydrate foods. Carbohydrates matter the most to you in your management of gestational diabetes. Many women find that they have difficulty eating too many carbohydrates in the morning and it causes them to have high blood sugar levels all day.
2. All foods contain some amount of carbohydrate, but your main concern is with food items that are <u>mainly</u> carbohydrate. Fat and protein are also going to affect your blood sugar, but not as quickly as carbohydrate. Your meal plan will help you stay on track.
3. Nutritious foods are important to your growing baby. Simple sugars (candy, sugar, sweets, dessert) are not very filling and don't contain a lot of nutritional value. Complex carbohydrates (whole grains, higher fiber foods) are full of vitamins, minerals and fiber and should be chosen more often.

4. Watch out for simple carbohydrates that raise your blood sugar quickly. Drinking regular fruit juices, regular sodas, kool-aid, and high sugar desserts like ice cream, pies and cookies all contribute to increasing your blood sugar quickly. When you read labels, look for the word "sugar" and keep it low. Ask your doctor or dietitian how much simple sugar you should eat per day.

5. Portion sizes are vitally important to how much your blood sugar changes. You can eat too much of healthy carbohydrate and raise your blood sugars too high. Your meal plan will tell you portion sizes and how many of them to eat—so try to watch how big your portions are and make sure you eat what you need without overeating. Choosing high fiber foods such as whole grain products and whole grain cereals, fresh and frozen vegetables, and beans are the best way to get your needed carbohydrates, and allows your body to absorb the carbohydrate over time.

6. What time you eat matters. In the morning, many women find that eating too many carbohydrate (more than 30 grams) makes their blood sugar really high. So you are better off to avoid juice and limit yourself to 2 portions of carbohydrate in the morning so you are in better control of your blood sugars all day. Eating a small breakfast, and another small snack a few hours later works well when this seems to be a problem.

7. Follow your meal plan to know how much to eat and when. A meal plan can help you allocate your food for the day and feel full without over eating. Eating 6 small meals tends to help the most with blood sugar control since you are asking your body to handle a smaller load of carbohydrate with each meal. Plan to eat about every 2-3 hours throughout the day to keep your blood sugars stable.

8. Check your blood sugars and document your intake. Good news! That is exactly what this book helps you do. You can track your meals, medications, blood sugars and how you are feeling for the day. Your doctor may have given you a meter, or you might just check your urine. Either way, following your meal plan and tracking your blood sugars helps a great deal to make you successful!

9. If you are gaining too much weight, look into how much fat is in the food you are eating. While fat won't immediately increase your blood sugar, it can add weight which is not always healthy for you or your baby. Try eating lean proteins—lean beef, chicken and fish that are grilled or baked instead of fried. Cut off the fat from meats before cooking, and always bake or grill your meats. Avoid fried foods if you can. And if you cannot, eat a much smaller portion of the food that was fried. Drink skim or low fat milk, and avoid adding extra butter or margarine. Eat less convenience foods and make more meals at home.

Label Reading For Gestational Diabetes

When you are shopping or cooking, notice that most food items have a "Nutrition Facts" label on them that tells you the amount of different nutrients the food contains. This label will help guide you in planning your meals.

The main thing to remember about a nutrition facts label is that it contains information on a per serving basis. So when you look at the carbohydrate and other amounts of nutrients, it is based on one serving. At the top of the label, you can see the size of a portion—and how many servings are in the container. So if you have a package that contains two servings, the amounts on the label should be doubled to get the correct calories, fat, protein and other nutrients if the entire container is eaten.

To figure out how many carbohydrate servings are in the food, you should look at the label and determine the standard serving size. This information is located at the top of the label. Then read the total grams of carbohydrate it contains per serving.

A single serving of carbohydrate is about 15 grams of carbohydrate. When you find the total grams of carbohydrate on the label, you should divide it by 15 to get the total number of servings of carbohydrate in one serving of the food item. You can ignore the total grams of sugar in this example because they are already included in the total grams of carbohydrate line. Once you know that number, you can understand how many servings of carbohydrate are in a single serving.

For example: if it contained 45 grams of carbohydrate in one serving of food, you would have 3 servings of carbohydrate per serving.

What Foods Have Carbohydrate?

Foods that contain carbohydrate in significant amounts that count for your meals are:

- Breads, crackers, and cereals
- Pasta, rice, and grains
- Starchy vegetables such as potatoes, corn, and peas
- Beans and legumes
- Milk, soy milk, and yogurt
- Fruits and fruit juices
- Regular sugar sweetened sodas
- Sweets, such as cakes, cookies, ice cream, jam and jelly

Starches are good sources of minerals, vitamins, and fiber when eating them as part of a healthy meal plan. Eating whole wheat bread, whole grain cereals (like oatmeal), and brown rice ensures you get more fiber in your diet. You should choose low fat, low salt and low sugar starches for the healthiest meals.

Fruits contain carbohydrate as well, and are good sources of vitamins A & C, minerals, and fiber. To make the most of these servings eat the peel from the fruit when you can, and avoid those made with additional sugars or sweeteners. In general, when you have gestational diabetes, you should avoid fruit juice because it may raise your blood sugar quickly. Eating whole fruit slows the absorption of the natural fruit sugars and makes them healthier for you and baby.

Milk products are a good source of protein, calcium, and vitamins A & D. Drinking nonfat or low-fat milk and yogurt products is a way to eat healthier without added fat. Make sure you stick with unsweetened versions of yogurt or soy milk to avoid added calories.

For non-starchy vegetables, you can eat about 1 cup of a raw vegetable or 1/2 cup of a cooked vegetable to get a low amount of carbohydrate. 1 cup of broccoli contains about 5 grams of carbohydrate. Non-starchy vegetables are good sources of vitamins and fiber. Preparing them without additional sauces and fats makes them very healthy—and sticking to the dark green leafy, orange, or yellow vegetables make the best choices.

Examples of carbohydrate serving sizes that equal 15 gm of carbohydrate

Starches

- 1 slice of bread (1 ounce)
- 1 tortilla
- 1/4 large bagel (1 ounce)
- 2 5-inch taco shells
- 1/2 hamburger or hot dog bun (1 ounce)
- 3/4 cup unsweetened cold cereal
- 4-6 crackers
- 1/3 cup pasta or rice (cooked)
- 1/2 cup beans, peas, corn, sweet potatoes, winter squash, or potatoes (cooked)
- 1/4 large baked potato (3 ounces)
- 3/4 ounce pretzels, potato or tortilla chips
- 3 cups popped popcorn

Fruit

- 1 small fresh fruit (4 ounces)
- 1/2 cup canned fruit
- 1/4 cup dried fruit (2 Tablespoons)
- 17 small grapes (3 ounces)
- 1 cup melon or berries
- 2 tablespoons raisins
- 1/2 cup fruit juice (4 ounces)

Milk

- 1 cup fat-free or reduced fat milk
- 1 cup soy milk
- 2/3 cup fat-free yogurt—plain or artificially sweetened (6 ounces)

Sweets and Desserts

- 2 inch square cake (unfrosted)
- 2 small cookies (2/3 ounce)
- 1/2 cup ice cream or frozen yogurt
- 1/4 cup sherbet or sorbet
- 1 tablespoon syrup, jam, jelly, table sugar or honey
- 2 tablespoons light syrup

Other Foods

- Count one cup raw vegetables or 1/2 cup cooked non-starchy vegetables as zero carbohydrate or "free" foods. If you eat 3 or more servings at one meal, count them as 1 carbohydrate serving
- Foods that have less than 20 calories in each serving are also counted as "free" foods.
- One cup of casserole dishes or other mixed foods count as 2 servings of carbohydrate

Proteins don't increase your blood sugar right away, but eating more protein increases your overall calories. Eating too many calories is not a good idea since it might increase your weight gain. Protein comes from meats and fish and is a good source of iron, zinc, and B vitamins. Trim off the excess fat from meats, choose low fat cheeses, eat more fish, and bake or broil instead of frying. While milk and beans contain protein, they fall under the carbohydrate choices since they contain about 15 grams of carbohydrate per ounce. Proteins are usually eaten by the ounce, and most of the time you should stick to about 3 ounces at a meal. (The size of a deck of cards.)

Fats help your body make hormones, provide flavor, and make foods taste good. You need some fat, but most people get more than enough. Choose unsaturated fats and oils most often to cook with—like olive or canola oil. Limit or avoid saturated fats—like those that are solid at room temperature (butter or margarine for example).

If you need some ideas for what amounts of portions of each type of food to eat on your meal plan, consider doing the following and watching your blood sugar carefully:

1. Vegetables—eat 6 or more servings of non-starchy vegetables that are fresh, frozen or canned. Non starchy vegetables are usually dark green, orange, or yellow. Potatoes, sweet potatoes, yams, peas, corn, and winter squash count as a grain/starch not as a vegetable. When you read a label, a non-starchy vegetable has 0-5 grams of carbohydrate per serving.
2. Protein—choose lean proteins and avoid bacon, hot dogs and fried meats. Daily, eat about 6 ounces of protein (more if your doctor tells you). Remember you get protein from many sources, but most sources of protein don't raise your blood sugar because they don't contain carbohydrate. Cheese counts as a protein, but beans are a starch. Try to consume about 2 servings per week of cooked fish.
3. Starches/Grains—Eat 100% whole grains, and avoid white starches like white rice,

noodles and potatoes. Make sure your foods contain fiber. Daily, aim for about 7 servings of starches/grains such as whole grain breads, tortillas, dried beans, pasta or rice. Each serving is about 15 grams of carbohydrate.

4. Fruits—Eating whole fruits is best. When you have gestational diabetes, it is recommended that you avoid fruit juice at all meals, and avoid fruit at breakfast. Try to eat 2 servings of fruit per day, and remember that one serving is 15 grams of carbohydrate.
5. Dairy—Eating pasteurized milk or yogurt is the only way to go! Choose about 3 servings of milk or yogurt daily during your pregnancy. Again, one serving equals about 15 grams of carbohydrate.
6. Fats and Oils—Limit this category to about 6 teaspoons per day, and use healthy plant oils like canola, olive and safflower oil for cooking. Read labels and avoid saturated fats or trans fats when you can.
7. Snacks—Snacks count in your overall plan and within the limits of your calories. Try to combine protein and starches at snacks to slow the absorption of carbohydrate and make you feel full longer. Eat about 2 hours apart, and drink plenty of water or other fluids.
8. Exercise—Don't forget to walk for about 10-15 minutes after a meal to control your blood sugars. Even if it's only around the block, you can make a difference in your blood sugar levels by walking.

On the next page is a blank meal pattern for you to use to plan out your day. Use pencil so that as your pregnancy progresses, you can change the pattern if need be. Wishing you the best with your pregnancy!

For my other books on gestational diabetes go to my Amazon Author Central Page at:

http://amazon.com/author/matheaford

Books are available on -

Gestational Diabetes Testing

How Gestational Diabetes Is Managed

Gestational Diabetes Meal Planning

I would love the chance to help you learn more about gestational diabetes and how to have a healthy pregnancy.

Note to the reader: Throughout the text we refer frequently to the woman (mother) and the baby (fetus). To help distinguish between the female role and the baby, we have decided that the baby is a boy. We understand that not all babies are male.

Mathea Ford, RD/LD

contact@healthydietmenusforyou.com

Gestational Diabetes Meal Pattern

Daily Target Amounts
Carbohydrate: ______________ grams per day (__________ Servings) [15 gm—1 serving]
Protein: ________________ grams per day (__________Servings)
Fat: _______________ grams per day (_____________Servings)
Calories: _________________

Write in your pattern for meals so you can reference it when you are documenting in the journal.

When	What and How Much
Breakfast At about _____ AM	Carbohydrates: ______ grams (___ servings) Starch _____ Milk_______ Fruit ______ Non-starchy vegetable ________ Protein: _______ grams (______ ounces) Fat: ______ grams (_______servings)
Mid Morning Snack At about _____ AM	Carbohydrates: ______ grams (___ servings) Starch _____ Milk_______ Fruit ______ Non-starchy vegetable ________ Protein: _______ grams (______ ounces) Fat: ______ grams (_______servings)
Lunch At about _____ AM/ PM	Carbohydrates: ______ grams (___ servings) Starch _____ Milk_______ Fruit ______ Non-starchy vegetable ________ Protein: _______ grams (______ ounces) Fat: ______ grams (_______servings)
Mid-Afternoon Snack At about ______ PM	Carbohydrates: ______ grams (___ servings) Starch _____ Milk_______ Fruit ______ Non-starchy vegetable ________ Protein: _______ grams (______ ounces) Fat: ______ grams (_______servings)
Dinner At about _______PM	Carbohydrates: ______ grams (___ servings) Starch _____ Milk_______ Fruit ______ Non-starchy vegetable ________ Protein: _______ grams (______ ounces) Fat: ______ grams (_______servings)
Evening Snack At about ______ PM	Carbohydrates: ______ grams (___ servings) Starch _____ Milk_______ Fruit ______ Non-starchy vegetable ________ Protein: _______ grams (______ ounces) Fat: ______ grams (_______servings)

Remember the starchy vegetables are: potatoes, corn, beans, and peas

How To Use Your Gestational Diabetes Journal

This is where you enter the date, weight, how much exercise you did, and any baby movements. You can also fill in how you feel, and your blood sugars.

Top of page tells you how many weeks and days pregnant you are. You enter day of week.

Today I am 24 Weeks and 1 Day Pregnant

Date: ______________________________ Day of Week: Su M T (W) Th F Sa

Morning Weight: ________________

Exercise: ____________________

Baby Movements or Activity:

____

Today I am

____

Because ________________________

____

Your daily information guide, tips about your baby are here!

Blood Sugar Tracking:

AM/Fasting: ________ After Lunch: ________

After Breakfast: ________ After Supper: ________

Blood Sugar Tracking—enter your numbers for the day

Morning	Carbs	Lunch	Carbs	Supper	Carbs	Snacks	Carbs

Enter your meals, and the amount of carbohydrate in the meal so you can track what you are eating!

Medications taken today:

Add the medications you took for the day so you can talk to your doctor about changes.

Today I am 24 Weeks and 1 Day Pregnant

Date: ______________________________ Day of Week: Su M T W Th F Sa

Morning Weight: __________________

Exercise: ______________________

Baby Movements or Activity:

____

Today I am

____

Because _____________________________

____

Nutrition Nugget: Calories

"Eating for two" doesn't mean you need to double up on calorie intake now that you're pregnant! But you do need a little extra every day – about 300 more calories per day than you typically consumed before pregnancy. Follow your meal pattern for your gestational diabetes and eat lots of colorful foods throughout the day. If you're exercising regularly, you may need more calories: if you're sedentary, you'll need fewer. The best diet is one full of whole foods, without many high-processed, high-fat, high-sugar foods. Try to eat a wide variety of foods, and get some protein, fats, carbohydrates, vitamins, and minerals in each meal or snack.

Blood Sugar Tracking:

AM/Fasting: _________ After Lunch: __________

After Breakfast: __________ After Supper: __________

Morning	Carbs	Lunch	Carbs	Supper	Carbs	Snacks	Carbs

Medications taken today:

Today I am 24 Weeks and 2 Days Pregnant

Date: ______________________________ Day of Week: Su M T W Th F Sa

Morning Weight: ____________________

Exercise: ____________________

Baby Movements or Activity:

____

Today I am

____

Because ______________________________

____

Blood Sugar Tracking:

AM/Fasting: ________ After Lunch: ________

After Breakfast: ________ After Supper: ________

Keeping Yourself Comfortable: Fatigue

Your body is working overtime growing a baby! One of the first pregnancy symptoms most women notice is fatigue. For most moms-to-be, the second trimester is filled with more energy. But by the third trimester, the fatigue starts to set in again. As obvious as it sounds, take time to rest every day – even if it's just a 20-minute power nap. Make sure you are eating well – six small meals a day should improve your energy levels. Keep yourself well hydrated – dehydration can lead to fatigue, headaches, and even contractions. Exercise will also give your flagging energy a boost.

Morning	Carbs	Lunch	Carbs	Supper	Carbs	Snacks	Carbs

Medications taken today:

Today I am 24 Weeks and 3 Days Pregnant

Date: ________________________________ Day of Week: Su M T W Th F Sa

Morning Weight: ____________________

Exercise: __________________________

Baby Movements or Activity:

____

Today I am

____

Because ____________________________

____

Blood Sugar Tracking:

AM/Fasting: ________ After Lunch: __________

After Breakfast: _________After Supper: __________

Oh Baby!

This week your baby is about the size of an ear of corn – 11 to 12 inches long and weighing a little more than a pound. He is floating in the amniotic fluid, which keeps him warm and cushions him from the outside world. The lungs are getting ready for breathing – a special protein is being produced that will keep them from sticking together when inhaling and exhaling. All of the other major organ systems are developed. The baby still needs some more time inside, though, to add fat to his body and to complete more growth and maturation.

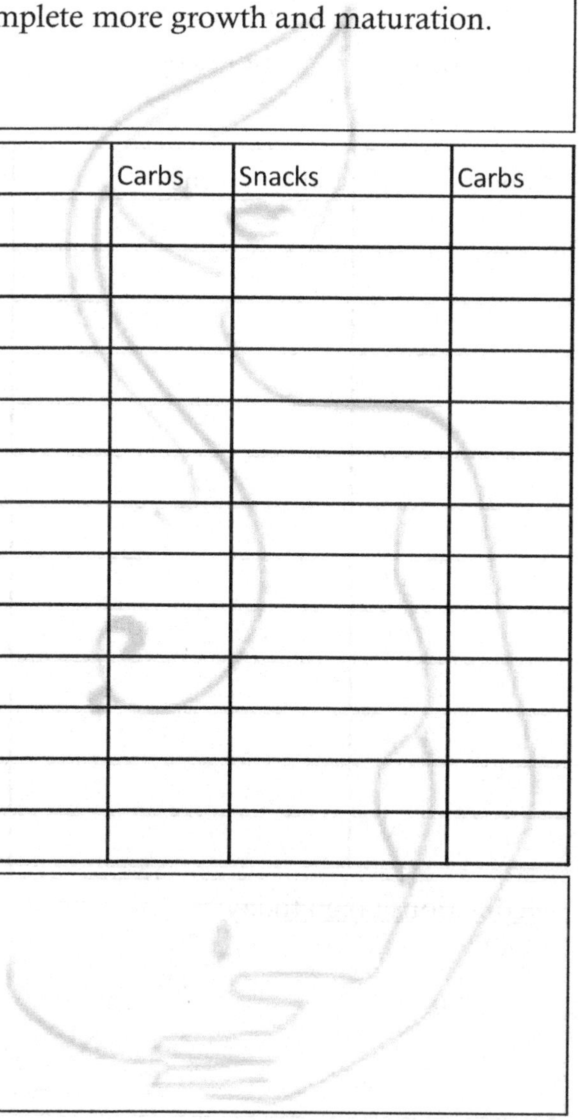

Morning	Carbs	Lunch	Carbs	Supper	Carbs	Snacks	Carbs

Medications taken today:

Today I am 24 Weeks and 4 Days Pregnant

Date: ______________________________ Day of Week: Su M T W Th F Sa

Morning Weight: __________________

Exercise: __________________

Baby Movements or Activity:

____

Today I am

____

Because ____________________________

____

Blood Sugar Tracking:

AM/Fasting: ________ After Lunch: __________

After Breakfast: _________After Supper: __________

Enjoyable Exercises: Tips for Starting Slow

If you didn't have a regular exercise program before getting pregnant, you may be wondering if you should try getting in shape now. Be sure to check with your healthcare provider before starting any new fitness program so you can be sure you don't have any limitations. "Snack" on exercise – add several short sessions throughout your day rather than one long session. Increase gradually – you don't need to run a marathon your first day out, try walking for 20-30 minutes instead. Avoid fatigue – if you get tired take a break or stop altogether. Keep yourself hydrated by drinking water before, during and after a workout. You may need a more supportive bra or an abdominal support to keep you comfortable in the later weeks of pregnancy.

Morning	Carbs	Lunch	Carbs	Supper	Carbs	Snacks	Carbs

Medications taken today:

Today I am 24 Weeks and 5 Days Pregnant

Date: ________________________________ Day of Week: Su M T W Th F Sa

Morning Weight: ____________________

Exercise: ____________________

Baby Movements or Activity:

____

Today I am

____

Because ____________________________

____

Blood Sugar Tracking:

AM/Fasting: ________ After Lunch: ________

After Breakfast: ________ After Supper: ________

Don't Forget the Dentist

The hormonal changes of pregnancy affect all of your body – including your gums and teeth. Many pregnant women notice bleeding gums when brushing and flossing. Experts think this isn't just hormones, but also the increased blood volume of pregnancy. Sometimes the gums get swollen, and small lumps may appear. These lumps aren't dangerous, but they may cause some discomfort. Women are at a greater risk of developing gingivitis (an infection of the gums) during pregnancy. Researchers have found that bacteria in your mouth might increase your risk of preterm labor, premature birth and low birth weight. Be sure to brush and floss every day, keep all regularly schedule teeth cleaning appointments, and call your dentist right away if you have any questions or problems.

Morning	Carbs	Lunch	Carbs	Supper	Carbs	Snacks	Carbs

Medications taken today:

Today I am 24 Weeks and 6 Days Pregnant

Date: ______________________________ Day of Week: Su M T W Th F Sa

Morning Weight: ____________________

Exercise: ____________________

Baby Movements or Activity:

____

Today I am

____

Because ________________________________

____

Blood Sugar Tracking:

AM/Fasting: _________ After Lunch: __________

After Breakfast: __________ After Supper: __________

Sex and Intimacy

Unless you have complications or are considered high-risk, sex is safe at all stages of a normal pregnancy. During the early months, fatigue and morning sickness may have made sex the furthest thing from your mind. But, in the second trimester, many women report a heightened libido. If you're feeling frisky, let your partner know. Some people worry that they will hurt the baby, or that the baby will somehow know what's going on. Don't let these myths limit your sex life. Don't feel like having intercourse? Find other ways to be intimate that don't involve penetration – massage, touching, even hand-holding can all be great ways to show your love for each other without having sex.

Morning	Carbs	Lunch	Carbs	Supper	Carbs	Snacks	Carbs

Medications taken today:

Today I am 24 Weeks and 7 Days Pregnant

Date: ______________________________ Day of Week: Su M T W Th F Sa

Morning Weight: __________________

Exercise: ______________________

Baby Movements or Activity:

____

Today I am

____

Because _____________________________

____

Blood Sugar Tracking:

AM/Fasting: ________ After Lunch: ________

After Breakfast: ________ After Supper: ________

Choosing Your Information Resources Wisely

Many books are published every year aimed at pregnant moms and dads. The Internet is rife with resources – some good, some less-than-helpful. How do you know which are the best? Ask friends and family who have recently given birth what their favorite resources were. If you read something that seems out of place, consult a few more sources to verify the truth. Internet videos can be a helpful way to see what happens during childbirth, but many aren't censored and can make you feel more scared. The same with television programs about birth, which tend to take the most sensational situations to air. While these can be entertaining to watch, keep in mind that birth is usually much more mundane - though it will still be a highlight of your life!

Morning	Carbs	Lunch	Carbs	Supper	Carbs	Snacks	Carbs

<u>Medications taken today:</u>

Overview Of My 24th Week:

Doctor's Visits Notes:

A Picture To Remember This Week

Today I am 25 Weeks and 1 Day Pregnant

Date: ______________________________ Day of Week: Su M T W Th F Sa

Morning Weight: ____________________

Exercise: ________________________

Baby Movements or Activity:

____

Today I am

____

Because ____________________________

____

Blood Sugar Tracking:

AM/Fasting: ________ After Lunch: ________

After Breakfast: ________ After Supper: ________

Nutrition Nugget: Portion Control

One of the best ways to keep from gaining too much weight during pregnancy is to keep your portions under control. Try using a salad plate rather than a dinner plate. Stop when you feel full, rather than continuing just because you still have food left on your plate. Chew slowly, and fully savor your food. These serving size comparison may help you keep from overeating:

3oz. of meat = deck of cards
Medium fruit = tennis ball
½ cup of ice cream = tennis ball
1 oz. cheese = 4 dice
1 cup of vegetables = size of your fist
1 tsp. butter or oil = size of the tip of your thumb

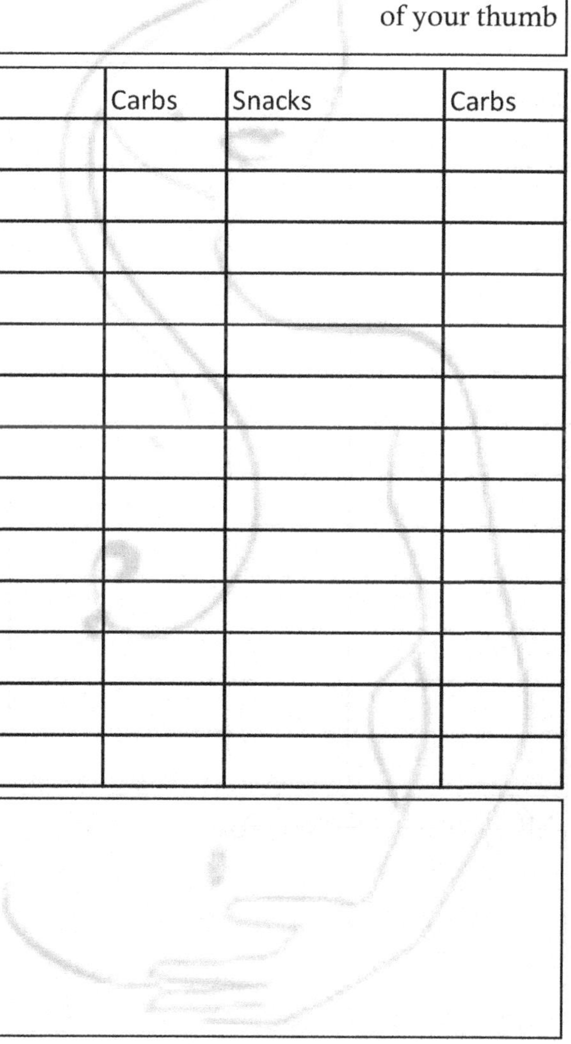

Morning	Carbs	Lunch	Carbs	Supper	Carbs	Snacks	Carbs

Medications taken today:

Today I am 25 Weeks and 2 Days Pregnant

Date: ______________________________ Day of Week: Su M T W Th F Sa

Morning Weight: ____________________

Exercise: ________________________

Baby Movements or Activity:

____

Today I am

____

Because ____________________________

____

Blood Sugar Tracking:

AM/Fasting: __________ After Lunch: __________

After Breakfast: __________After Supper: __________

Keeping Yourself Comfortable: Headaches and Dizziness

Occasional dizziness is normal in pregnancy, especially when you change positions such as moving to sitting from lying down. The culprit is your increased blood volume along with hormones relaxing the blood vessels. Dizziness can also stem from low blood sugar. Headaches are also common and can also be blamed on hormones and increased blood volume. Other factors, such as low blood sugar, dehydration and stress can contribute, as well. You can try to prevent headaches by getting enough sleep, eating well, staying hydrated, exercising regularly, and practicing good posture. If you ever feel dizzy at rest, if you faint, if your headaches don't go away easily, if they start happening more often or if they are accompanied by blurred vision, sudden weight gain, or unusual swelling in the hands and face, let your provider know right away.

Morning	Carbs	Lunch	Carbs	Supper	Carbs	Snacks	Carbs

Medications taken today:

Today I am 25 Weeks and 3 Days Pregnant

Date: ______________________________ Day of Week: Su M T W Th F Sa

Morning Weight: __________________

Exercise: ________________________

Baby Movements or Activity:

____

Today I am

____

Because ___________________________

____

Oh Baby!

Your baby is about the size of a papaya this week, measuring 13.5 inches long and weighing about 1.5 pounds. The bone centers are starting to harden, and the spine with all of its intricacies (including 33 vertebrae, 150 joints, and 1,000 ligaments) is developed. All of the tiny details of the hands and fingers are complete. Brain waves start to emerge, and your baby's little brain may be able to remember things like the sound of your voice or the music you play often. Your baby even has a startle reflex – and he may shield his ears with his beautiful little hands.

Blood Sugar Tracking:

AM/Fasting: ________ After Lunch: __________

After Breakfast: __________After Supper: __________

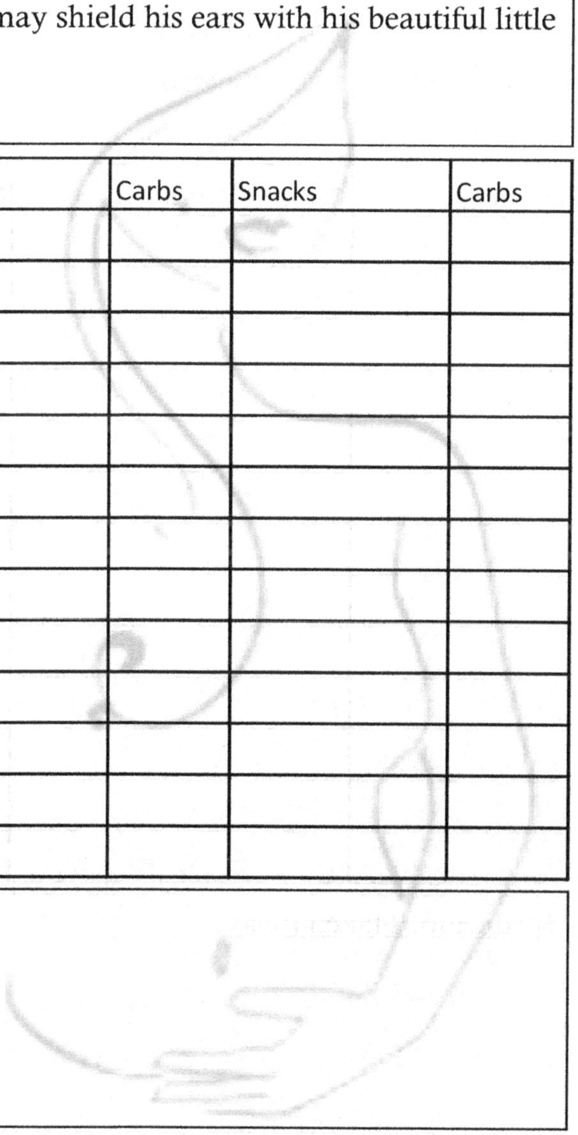

Morning	Carbs	Lunch	Carbs	Supper	Carbs	Snacks	Carbs

<u>Medications taken today:</u>

Today I am 25 Weeks and 4 Days Pregnant

Date: ______________________________ Day of Week: Su M T W Th F Sa

Morning Weight: __________________

Exercise: __________________

Baby Movements or Activity:

____

Today I am

____

Because ______________________________

____

Blood Sugar Tracking:

AM/Fasting: ________ After Lunch: ________

After Breakfast: ________ After Supper: ________

Enjoyable Exercises: Stretching

Stretching exercises can relieve back pain, strengthen leg and abdominal muscles, and help to prepare your body for childbirth. Try tailor sitting: sit on the floor, bend your knees and cross your ankles. As you get comfortable, lean forward, letting your baby belly drop between your legs. Or work on pressing your knees toward the floor. Squatting provides another great stretch. Keep your knees wider than your hips, and allow your bottom to fall toward the floor. You may need to lean your body forward with your belly between your legs, and you may need something to hold onto nearby. Hold the squat briefly, and then allow yourself to sit down.

Morning	Carbs	Lunch	Carbs	Supper	Carbs	Snacks	Carbs

Medications taken today:

Today I am 25 Weeks and 5 Days Pregnant

Date: ______________________________ Day of Week: Su M T W Th F Sa

Morning Weight: ________________

Exercise: ________________

Baby Movements or Activity:

____

Today I am

____

Because ______________________________

____

Blood Sugar Tracking:

AM/Fasting: ________ After Lunch: ________

After Breakfast: ________ After Supper: ________

Controlling Cravings

Possibly the most joked-about aspect of pregnancy, cravings and aversions happen to the majority of pregnant women at some point. Sometimes foods you rarely eat become foods you can't get enough of! While cravings are probably harmless make sure they don't interfere with proper nutrition. Try for healthy alternatives. Craving sweets? Try fruit instead of chocolate or cookies. Craving salty? Instead of chips, try roasted sweet potato fries. If you are craving non-food items (called *pica*), get help from your healthcare provider and learn how to deal with this issue. It's not uncommon to have aversions to foods and smells, too. Your sense of smell and taste generally return to normal after the first trimester, and aversions tend to dissipate then.

Morning	Carbs	Lunch	Carbs	Supper	Carbs	Snacks	Carbs

Medications taken today:

Today I am 25 Weeks and 6 Days Pregnant

Date: ______________________________ Day of Week: Su M T W Th F Sa

Morning Weight: ____________________

Exercise: ________________________

Baby Movements or Activity:

____

Today I am

____

Because ___________________________

____

Blood Sugar Tracking:

AM/Fasting: ________ After Lunch: ________

After Breakfast: ________ After Supper: ________

Weight gain: Where Does the Weight Go?

Ever wonder where all that weight you're gaining is going? Here's a breakdown of how pregnancy weight is distributed by the time you deliver: your baby will be, on average, 7 pounds; the placenta typically weighs about 1.5 pounds; the amniotic fluid and the uterus, about 2 pounds each; your breasts will have gained about 2 pounds and your body will have gained 4 pounds each of blood and fluid. You will add some fat stores as well – 7 pounds on average – to be used by your body in the postpartum. Keep in mind, this isn't just getting fat – it's growing a baby. Weight gain to be excited about!

Morning	Carbs	Lunch	Carbs	Supper	Carbs	Snacks	Carbs

Medications taken today:

Today I am 25 Weeks and 7 Days Pregnant

Date: ______________________________ Day of Week: Su M T W Th F Sa

Morning Weight: __________________

Exercise: ______________________

Baby Movements or Activity:

____

Today I am

____

Because ____________________________

____

Blood Sugar Tracking:

AM/Fasting: ________ After Lunch: ________

After Breakfast: ________ After Supper: ________

Baby's developing senses

A baby's senses develop rapidly during pregnancy, and are all in place at the time of birth. The sense of smell is the first to develop, and taste buds are in place by week 18. Your baby can actually taste and smell the your foods in the amniotic fluid. The ears begin to stand out on the sides of baby's head around week 18, and your baby can then hear you! By birth, he will be able to recognize voices – especially those of your partner or any siblings, even the family dog. The eyelids open around week 27 so that baby can see the dim womb environment. Vision will be refined after birth. Touch is well developed from very early in pregnancy, so your baby can likely feel you rubbing your tummy.

Morning	Carbs	Lunch	Carbs	Supper	Carbs	Snacks	Carbs

Medications taken today:

Overview Of My 25th Week:

Doctor's Visits Notes:

A Picture To Remember This Week

Today I am 26 Weeks and 1 Day Pregnant

Date: ______________________________ Day of Week: Su M T W Th F Sa

Morning Weight: ________________

Exercise: ________________

Baby Movements or Activity:

____

Today I am

____

Because ______________________________

____

Blood Sugar Tracking:

AM/Fasting: ________ After Lunch: ________

After Breakfast: ________ After Supper: ________

Nutrition Nugget: Carbohydrates

Carbohydrates should make up the largest part of your diet, and it's best if they are complex carbs rather than simple carbs. Complex carbs are those found in whole grains and plant foods that provide your body with long-lasting energy. The recommendation is that 40% to 50% of your total daily calories should come from complex carbs. Simple carbohydrates come from sugar and glucose sources and provide short bursts of energy, but can lead to cravings and binge eating. Carbohydrates will also provide you with many vitamins and minerals as well as much-needed fiber. A serving size of carbohydrates is about ½ to 1 cup, depending on the food source.

Morning	Carbs	Lunch	Carbs	Supper	Carbs	Snacks	Carbs

Medications taken today:

Today I am 26 Weeks and 2 Days Pregnant

Date: ______________________________ Day of Week: Su M T W Th F Sa

Morning Weight: __________________

Exercise: __________________

Baby Movements or Activity:

____

Today I am

____

Because _________________________________

____

Blood Sugar Tracking:

AM/Fasting: _________ After Lunch: __________

After Breakfast: __________ After Supper: __________

Keeping Yourself Comfortable: Swelling

Swelling of your hands and feet is pretty common in pregnancy. Increasing the amount of potassium in your diet, as well as decreasing the amount of salt and caffeine you consume, may help prevent swelling. Other ways to relieve swelling include swimming, increasing your fluids, and elevating your feet as often as you can. Sometimes support hose are recommended, but try to dress in loose clothing as much as possible, and try to avoid wearing high-heeled shoes. Sometimes swelling indicates a health problem, so let your doctor know about any unusual swelling right away, especially if it happens in your face, or if it is accompanied by other symptoms, such as blurred vision or headaches.

Morning	Carbs	Lunch	Carbs	Supper	Carbs	Snacks	Carbs

Medications taken today:

Today I am 26 Weeks and 3 Days Pregnant

Date: ______________________________ Day of Week: Su M T W Th F Sa

Morning Weight: ____________________

Exercise: ____________________

Baby Movements or Activity:

____

Today I am

____

Because ______________________________

____

Blood Sugar Tracking:

AM/Fasting: ________ After Lunch: ________

After Breakfast: ________ After Supper: ________

Oh Baby!

Your baby is around 14 inches long at this point in pregnancy – like a bunch of celery. Your baby's eyes are fully developed by now, and begin to open this week. He may even react if you shine a flash-light onto the belly and into his womb-home. Brain growth is the highlight over the coming weeks, with most of your baby's energy going to this function. Your baby is putting on more fat, though that won't be completed until closer to birth. Your baby is practicing breathing with amniotic fluid rather than air, and is practicing sucking – maybe even on his thumbs or fingers.

Morning	Carbs	Lunch	Carbs	Supper	Carbs	Snacks	Carbs

Medications taken today:

Today I am 26 Weeks and 4 Days Pregnant

Date: ______________________________ Day of Week: Su M T W Th F Sa

Morning Weight: __________________

Exercise: ______________________

Baby Movements or Activity:

____

Today I am

____

Because _____________________________

____

Blood Sugar Tracking:

AM/Fasting: _______ After Lunch: _______

After Breakfast: _______ After Supper: _______

Enjoyable Exercises: Swimming

Swimming is one of the best exercises for pregnancy, especially as your baby bump gets larger. Having your body surrounded on all sides by water supports your muscles and joints, helping you avoid injury and feel less fatigued. Swimming gives you a great aerobic workout, strengthening your muscles, including your heart. When your blood is circulating and flowing properly, nutrients are delivered more efficiently to your baby, and both mom and baby get more oxygen. Swimming can also keep you from overheating during exercise. Other benefits include relief from back pain, better sleep, and even decreased swelling in your feet and ankles.

Morning	Carbs	Lunch	Carbs	Supper	Carbs	Snacks	Carbs

Medications taken today:

Today I am 26 Weeks and 5 Days Pregnant

Date: ______________________________ Day of Week: Su M T W Th F Sa

Morning Weight: __________________

Exercise: __________________

Baby Movements or Activity:

____

Today I am

____

Because ______________________________

____

Blood Sugar Tracking:

AM/Fasting: ________ After Lunch: ________

After Breakfast: ________ After Supper: ________

Pregnancy dreams

Many women claim they have more vivid dreams during pregnancy than ever before. Some women have realistic dreams, or even nightmares, about caring for their baby. All moms wonder if these tales are their subconscious trying to tell them something. Scientists still don't understand why we dream – pregnant or not – but they do believe dreaming is a natural way for your mind to work through anxiety and worry. Rather than worrying that your dreams foretell future disasters, talk to someone you trust about what's bothering you. Try keeping a dream diary during pregnancy, which can make a great keepsake and may help you work through any fears you may have.

Morning	Carbs	Lunch	Carbs	Supper	Carbs	Snacks	Carbs

Medications taken today:

Today I am 26 Weeks and 6 Days Pregnant

Date: ______________________________ Day of Week: Su M T W Th F Sa

Morning Weight: ________________

Exercise: ________________

Baby Movements or Activity:

____

Today I am

____

Because ____________________________

____

Blood Sugar Tracking:

AM/Fasting: ________ After Lunch: ________

After Breakfast: ________ After Supper: ________

Lifestyle: Dieting During Pregnancy?

Most doctors do not recommend dieting during pregnancy, even if you were overweight when you conceived. Dieting is essentially starving yourself so that your body uses its fat stores for energy, helping you lose weight. But you certainly don't want to starve your growing baby. Eating a well-balanced diet with a variety of foods will help your baby grow and will keep you feeling good without gaining excessive amounts of weight. After your baby is born, you will have plenty of time to lose weight – breastfeeding may even help (another great reason to plan to nurse your baby).

Morning	Carbs	Lunch	Carbs	Supper	Carbs	Snacks	Carbs

Medications taken today:

Today I am 26 Weeks and 7 Days Pregnant

Date: ________________________________ Day of Week: Su M T W Th F Sa

Morning Weight: ____________________

Exercise: ____________________

Baby Movements or Activity:

____

Today I am

____

Because ________________________________

____

Blood Sugar Tracking:

AM/Fasting: ________ After Lunch: ________

After Breakfast: ________ After Supper: ________

Is This Medicine Safe?

Before you take any medication, whether it's an over-the-counter cold remedy, an herbal preparation for illness, or a dietary supplement, be sure to check with your doctor. If you were taking medication for a chronic condition before pregnancy, it's important to discuss this with your healthcare provider. Certain medications in pregnancy are known to cause birth defects, and your doctor can let you know whether something is safe, if an alternative would be better, or if taking nothing is the best choice. Only take a medication if the benefit outweighs any risk, and keep in mind that no drug is 100% safe. Finding non-drug comfort measures may be a better option.

Morning	Carbs	Lunch	Carbs	Supper	Carbs	Snacks	Carbs

Medications taken today:

Overview Of My 26th Week:

Doctor's Visits Notes:

A Picture To Remember This Week

Today I am 27 Weeks and 1 Day Pregnant

Date: ______________________________ Day of Week: Su M T W Th F Sa

Morning Weight: __________________

Exercise: ______________________

Baby Movements or Activity:

____

Today I am

____

Because ____________________________

____

Blood Sugar Tracking:

AM/Fasting: ________ After Lunch: ________

After Breakfast: ________ After Supper: ________

Nutrition Nugget: Fiber

Fiber is an important part of a balanced diet whether you're pregnant or not. Your daily requirements for fiber increase during pregnancy - you need 25 grams per day. Fiber can keep you from getting constipated, and can lower your blood pressure. Soluble fiber keeps you feeling fuller longer, and keeps you from large fluctuations in your blood sugar. Good food sources are oats, beans, lentils, and some fruits. Insoluble fiber helps move materials through the intestines, and includes whole grains, nuts, bran fiber, fruit skins, and many vegetables. Eat a varied combination of these foods each day for the best effect.

Morning	Carbs	Lunch	Carbs	Supper	Carbs	Snacks	Carbs

Medications taken today:

Today I am 27 Weeks and 2 Days Pregnant

Date: ______________________ Day of Week: Su M T W Th F Sa

Morning Weight: ______________

Exercise: ______________

Baby Movements or Activity:

____

Today I am

____

Because ______________________

____

Blood Sugar Tracking:

AM/Fasting: ________ After Lunch: ________

After Breakfast: ________ After Supper: ________

Keeping Yourself Comfortable: Constipation

During pregnancy, the hormone progesterone slows the digestive tract, which can lead to constipation. Prenatal vitamin supplements can also add to it, especially if they contain extra iron. The best ways to treat constipation are to eat more fiber, and to drink plenty of water (at least eight glasses per day). Some fruits and fruit juices (especially prune) may help to soften your stool and make having a bowel movement easier. Try using a footstool when you are trying to pass a bowel movement – it puts your legs into a squatting position that may make going easier. Regular exercise every day is a great prevention strategy, as is avoiding foods that tend to constipate.

Morning	Carbs	Lunch	Carbs	Supper	Carbs	Snacks	Carbs

Medications taken today:

Today I am 27 Weeks and 3 Days Pregnant

Date: ______________________________ Day of Week: Su M T W Th F Sa

Morning Weight: __________________

Exercise: _______________________

Baby Movements or Activity:

____

Today I am

____

Because _____________________________

____

Blood Sugar Tracking:

AM/Fasting: _________ After Lunch: __________

After Breakfast: _________ After Supper: __________

Oh Baby!

By this week – the last week of your second trimester – your baby is nearly fifteen inches long from head to toe, and weighs just over two pounds. He is about the size of a head of cauliflower. Your baby is moving more than ever, taking advantage of still having extra space inside the womb. The little one's even got sleeping and waking patterns. He is lulled to sleep by rocking, so you may notice less movement when you're busy during the day. At night when you slow down, though, your little one may wake up and practice all his movement skills.

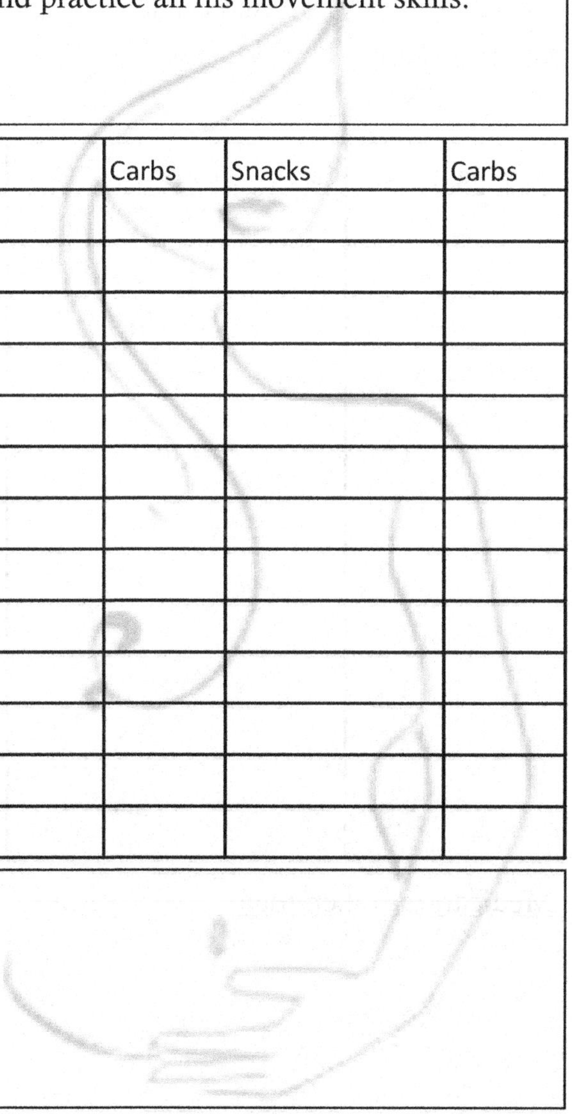

Morning	Carbs	Lunch	Carbs	Supper	Carbs	Snacks	Carbs

Medications taken today:

Today I am 27 Weeks and 4 Days Pregnant

Date: ______________________________ Day of Week: Su M T W Th F Sa

Morning Weight: __________________

Exercise: ________________________

Baby Movements or Activity:

____

Today I am

____

Because ___________________________

____

Blood Sugar Tracking:

AM/Fasting: ________ After Lunch: ________

After Breakfast: ________ After Supper: ________

Enjoyable Exercises: Yoga

The gentle movements of yoga may seem like stretching and relaxation, but yoga can, in fact, give you quite a workout! During pregnancy, try to find a class specifically for pregnant women. When choosing a yoga class, be sure to ask about the instructor's qualifications, and find out if he or she is certified or has additional training to work with prenatal clients. If the class is not set up for prenatal members, ask if they instructor is comfortable and knowledgeable about modifying poses for a pregnant mom. The benefits of yoga go beyond physical conditioning. Meditation and breathing practice – a part of most prenatal sessions – will give you relaxation skills you can rely on in childbirth.

Morning	Carbs	Lunch	Carbs	Supper	Carbs	Snacks	Carbs

Medications taken today:

Today I am 27 Weeks and 5 Days Pregnant

Date: ______________________________ Day of Week: Su M T W Th F Sa

Morning Weight: ____________________

Exercise: ____________________

Baby Movements or Activity:

____

Today I am

____

Because ______________________________

____

Choosing a birthing class

Just learning more about birth can help you feel less fearful and more prepared for the coming event. Many hospitals offer classes, and some areas have independent instructors. You may hear the words Lamaze, Bradley, Hypnobirthing, and more. These titles all describe different approaches to the birth process, with some overlap in what topics are covered in classes. Most childbirth preparation classes discuss normal birth, comfort measures for labor, labor positions, labor complications, medications, postpartum recovery, and more. Another important aspect of birthing classes is preparing the birth partner – so this is definitely something you can do as a couple to get ready for labor and the birth of your baby.

Blood Sugar Tracking:

AM/Fasting: ________ After Lunch: ________

After Breakfast: ________ After Supper: ________

Morning	Carbs	Lunch	Carbs	Supper	Carbs	Snacks	Carbs

Medications taken today:

Today I am 27 Weeks and 6 Days Pregnant

Date: ______________________________ Day of Week: Su M T W Th F Sa

Morning Weight: ____________________

Exercise: ________________________

Baby Movements or Activity:

____

Today I am

____

Because ___________________________

____

Blood Sugar Tracking:

AM/Fasting: ________ After Lunch: ________

After Breakfast: ________ After Supper: ________

Weight Gain Basics

While too much weight gain can make labor and delivery more challenging, gaining too little might cause growth and development problems for your baby. A pregnant woman typically gains 25 to 35 pounds by the time her baby is born. This recommendation depends on your pre-pregnant body size, though. (If you were underweight before pregnancy you will need to gain more. If you were overweight, you should gain a little less.) This weight gain will vary during a pregnancy, too. During the first trimester, a woman generally only gains about 2 to 4 pounds total. But for the remainder of pregnancy, a woman should gain about 1 pound a week.

Morning	Carbs	Lunch	Carbs	Supper	Carbs	Snacks	Carbs

Medications taken today:

Today I am 27 Weeks and 7 Days Pregnant

Date: ______________________________ Day of Week: Su M T W Th F Sa

Morning Weight: __________________

Exercise: __________________

Baby Movements or Activity:

____

Today I am

____

Because ______________________________

____

Blood Sugar Tracking:

AM/Fasting: ________ After Lunch: ________

After Breakfast: ________ After Supper: ________

Consider a Blessingway

While a traditional baby shower will help you accumulate much of the baby gear you want or need, a blessingway can be a great approach to honor your transition to motherhood. A blessingway can be adapted to any religious or cultural beliefs, it can be as long or as short as you would like, and it can be tailored to your individual style. The most important element should be pampering the mother-to-be with massage, hair brushing, or even body art. Storytelling and feasting are two other common features. If guests want to bring gifts, make them symbolic, such as something the mom can take with her in labor or a keepsake she can pass down to her child. Be creative!

Morning	Carbs	Lunch	Carbs	Supper	Carbs	Snacks	Carbs

Medications taken today:

Overview Of My 27th Week:

Doctor's Visits Notes:

A Picture To Remember This Week

Today I am 28 Weeks and 1 Day Pregnant

Date: ______________________________ Day of Week: Su M T W Th F Sa

Morning Weight: __________________

Exercise: __________________

Baby Movements or Activity:

____

Today I am

____

Because ______________________________

____

Blood Sugar Tracking:

AM/Fasting: _________ After Lunch: __________

After Breakfast: __________ After Supper: __________

Nutrition Nugget: "Complete" Meals and Snacks

Make the most of each and every meal by being sure to pack a nutritional punch while limiting excess calories. A "complete" meal is one containing a fat, a carbohydrate and a protein. By making sure these three elements are contained in any food combination you eat, you will maintain your blood sugar, keep your weight gain stable, and keep yourself feeling fuller longer. For instance, peanut butter on wheat bread with a glass of milk makes a great complete snack. Or how about chicken salad with some apple chunks in a whole grain pita? Follow your gestational diabetes meal plan and make sure you eat your meals and snacks to keep your baby growing.

Morning	Carbs	Lunch	Carbs	Supper	Carbs	Snacks	Carbs

Medications taken today:

Today I am 28 Weeks and 2 Days Pregnant

Date: ______________________________ Day of Week: Su M T W Th F Sa

Morning Weight: __________________

Exercise: ______________________

Baby Movements or Activity:

____

Today I am

____

Because ____________________________

____

Blood Sugar Tracking:

AM/Fasting: _________ After Lunch: __________

After Breakfast: _________ After Supper: __________

Keeping Yourself Comfortable: Back Ache

Backache is likely the most common complaint of the third trimester. As your baby and uterus grow, your center of gravity is pulled forward taking your lower back with it. For relief, pay close attention to your posture - imagine a string pulling your head up like a marionette, stretching and straightening your back. Practice proper body mechanics – bending at the knees not the waist, carrying heavy items close to your body. Do some stretching exercises. Consider using a warm heating pad on your lower back – you can even make one yourself! Place 2 pounds of white rice (not instant) in an old sock, tie it shut, and warm in the microwave for 2-3 minutes. You can even add some aromatherapy oil to this reusable comfort tool.

Morning	Carbs	Lunch	Carbs	Supper	Carbs	Snacks	Carbs

Medications taken today:

Today I am 28 Weeks and 3 Days Pregnant

Date: ______________________________ Day of Week: Su M T W Th F Sa

Morning Weight: __________________

Exercise: ____________________

Baby Movements or Activity:

____

Today I am

____

Because ______________________________

____

Oh Baby!

Welcome to the third trimester! At the size of an eggplant, your baby still has a lot of growing to do. He's now just over 15 inches long, and may weigh as much as 2.5 pounds. From here on out, your baby's body is gaining fat and muscle, while his brain continues to grow neurons and make connections. He also exhibits REM (rapid eye movement) during sleep. In adults, this is associated with dreaming, so it could mean some dreams for your baby, too. Blood vessels are forming throughout both of your baby's lungs and the bronchial tubes are dividing into branches, getting ready for breathing air rather than amniotic fluid.

Blood Sugar Tracking:

AM/Fasting: ________ After Lunch: ________

After Breakfast: ________ After Supper: ________

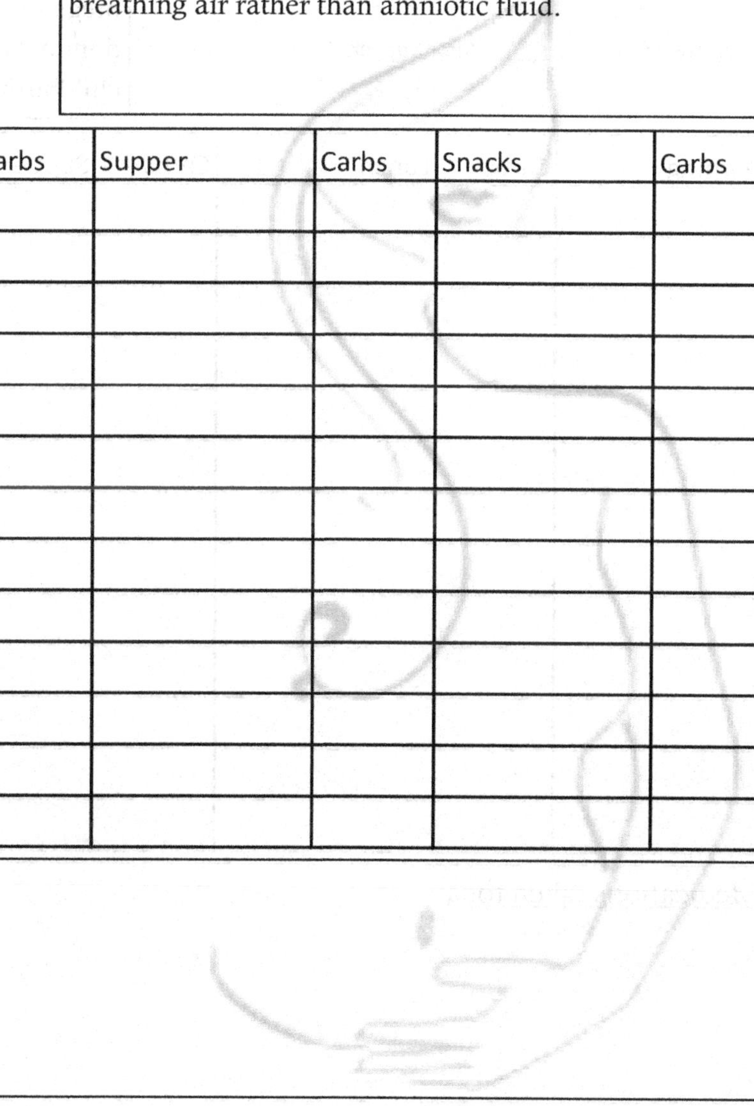

Morning	Carbs	Lunch	Carbs	Supper	Carbs	Snacks	Carbs

Medications taken today:

Today I am 28 Weeks and 4 Days Pregnant

Date: ______________________________ Day of Week: Su M T W Th F Sa

Morning Weight: ____________________

Exercise: __________________________

Baby Movements or Activity:

____

Today I am

____

Because ______________________________

____

Blood Sugar Tracking:

AM/Fasting: ________ After Lunch: ________

After Breakfast: ________ After Supper: ________

Enjoyable Exercises: Dance

Middle Eastern dance, or belly dancing, is an ancient tradition to prepare women for birth. You don't need to practice belly dancing; any type of dance will provide you with many benefits. Dance is a great way to maintain overall fitness, since it works many large muscle groups at the same time. It improves balance and coordination, which is sometimes impacted by the change in your center of gravity as your baby grows. As an aerobic exercise, it stimulates the circulatory system and breathing, improving oxygenation for both mom and baby. It promotes good posture, and can relieve backache during pregnancy. Belly dancing, specifically, can improve abdominal control and pelvic floor tone, preparing you for childbirth.

Morning	Carbs	Lunch	Carbs	Supper	Carbs	Snacks	Carbs

Medications taken today:

Today I am 28 Weeks and 5 Days Pregnant

Date: ______________________________ Day of Week: Su M T W Th F Sa

Morning Weight: __________________

Exercise: ___________________

Baby Movements or Activity:

____

Today I am

____

Because ___________________________

____

Pregnancy Skin Care

You've heard about the glowing skin of pregnancy, but you're looking in the mirror wondering when and if it's going to happen for you. Skin color changes are common in pregnancy. Some women suffer from dark patches of skin, called chloasma or the "mask of pregnancy." Others have itchiness, especially around the belly. Acne is also a common problem for pregnant women. The linea nigra – a dark line on the abdomen – may show up any time now, as may stretch marks. Most of these skin changes are caused by pregnancy hormones, and will likely disappear or lighten shortly after delivery. For now, using natural moisturizers and keeping your skin clean is the best way of treating these annoyances.

Blood Sugar Tracking:

AM/Fasting: _________ After Lunch: _________

After Breakfast: _________ After Supper: _________

Morning	Carbs	Lunch	Carbs	Supper	Carbs	Snacks	Carbs

Medications taken today:

Today I am 28 Weeks and 6 Days Pregnant

Date: ______________________ Day of Week: Su M T W Th F Sa

Morning Weight: ______________

Exercise: ______________

Baby Movements or Activity:

____

Today I am

____

Because ______________________

____

Blood Sugar Tracking:

AM/Fasting: ________ After Lunch: ________

After Breakfast: ________ After Supper: ________

Lifestyle: Caffeine and Pregnancy

Researchers suggest that pregnant women (and women trying to conceive) limit their caffeine intake to 200 milligrams per day – the amount in about 12 ounces of coffee. Take into consideration all caffeine sources when you consider your diet – coffee, tea, soda, chocolate. And keep in mind the amount of caffeine varies. Coffee, for instance, has different levels depending on how it's prepared, what types of beans are used, and the way it is served. Caffeine can decrease blood flow in the placenta, and it does cross over to your baby's body, though the long-term effects aren't known.

Morning	Carbs	Lunch	Carbs	Supper	Carbs	Snacks	Carbs

Medications taken today:

Today I am 28 Weeks and 7 Days Pregnant

Date: ______________________________ Day of Week: Su M T W Th F Sa

Morning Weight: ____________________

Exercise: ____________________

Baby Movements or Activity:

____

Today I am

____

Because ______________________________

____

Pregnancy Traditions: Seven-Month Ceremonies

In a variety of cultures around the world, the seventh month of pregnancy is celebrated with a feast or ceremony to mark the new life inside. You can plan your own celebration to honor your active baby and your coming motherhood. In Guatemala, mothers describe everyday scenes aloud to her unborn baby. You might walk around your home or neighborhood and do the same. You could introduce your baby to family by looking through photos and telling your memories about the events. This is a great way to bond with your unborn child. Most importantly, incorporate a feast into your celebration and be sure to include all the special people in your life.

Blood Sugar Tracking:

AM/Fasting: _________ After Lunch: _________

After Breakfast: _________After Supper: _________

Morning	Carbs	Lunch	Carbs	Supper	Carbs	Snacks	Carbs

Medications taken today:

Overview Of My 28th Week:

Doctor's Visits Notes:

A Picture To Remember This Week

Today I am 29 Weeks and 1 Day Pregnant

Date: ______________________________ Day of Week: Su M T W Th F Sa

Morning Weight: __________________

Exercise: __________________

Baby Movements or Activity:

____

Today I am

____

Because ______________________________

____

Blood Sugar Tracking:

AM/Fasting: ________ After Lunch: ________

After Breakfast: ________ After Supper: ________

Nutrition Nugget: Protein

During the second and third trimester, your baby's major systems are in place, and huge leaps in growth begin to happen. Protein provides the building blocks your body and your baby's body need for this growth and development. A pregnant woman typically needs about 70 grams of protein each day, which can be achieved in about three or four servings of protein-rich foods (one serving is about the size of a deck of cards). Good sources of protein include lean meat, poultry, and fish; eggs; milk and milk products; and, beans, nuts and legumes. If you are a vegetarian, getting enough protein might be challenging, so be sure to add enough dairy, soy and beans to your diet.

Morning	Carbs	Lunch	Carbs	Supper	Carbs	Snacks	Carbs

Medications taken today:

Today I am 29 Weeks and 2 Days Pregnant

Date: ______________________ Day of Week: Su M T W Th F Sa

Morning Weight: ______________

Exercise: ______________

Baby Movements or Activity:

____

Today I am

____

Because ______________________

____

Blood Sugar Tracking:

AM/Fasting: ________ After Lunch: ________

After Breakfast: ________ After Supper: ________

Tips for Sleeping Comfortably

It can be hard to get a good night's sleep when you're pregnant – finding a comfortable position is near impossible, and you keep waking anyway to use the bathroom. Try taking a warm bath before bed to relax your body. Perhaps your partner can give you a pre-slumber massage. Use extra pillows to support your back, belly and legs. Consider a mug of warm decaffeinated tea or warm milk before you go to bed. If heartburn is waking you, you may need to sleep propped up on several pillows. Your grandma may suggest a cup of warm milk or chamomile tea to help you sleep – just make sure you have it an hour or so before you plan to go to bed so you don't keep waking to use the bathroom.

Morning	Carbs	Lunch	Carbs	Supper	Carbs	Snacks	Carbs

Medications taken today:

Today I am 29 Weeks and 3 Days Pregnant

Date: ______________________________ Day of Week: Su M T W Th F Sa

Morning Weight: ____________________

Exercise: ________________________

Baby Movements or Activity:

____

Today I am

____

Because ___________________________

____

Blood Sugar Tracking:

AM/Fasting: ________ After Lunch: ________

After Breakfast: ________ After Supper: ________

Oh Baby!

Now about the size of a head of lettuce, your baby weighs around 2.75 pounds, and measures about 15.5 inches from head to toe. Over the remainder of your pregnancy as more subcutaneous fat is laid down, your baby will double or triple in weight. His skin is getting less translucent, and losing many of its folds. Temperature regulation is a huge milestone this week. Your baby's body is learning to maintain a comfy 101°F/ 38.5°C. Your baby still needs the warmth of your body, though, and will even after birth. His head is growing to accommodate the expanding brain, where hundreds of billions of brain cells are developing.

Morning	Carbs	Lunch	Carbs	Supper	Carbs	Snacks	Carbs

Medications taken today:

Today I am 29 Weeks and 4 Days Pregnant

Date: ______________________________ Day of Week: Su M T W Th F Sa

Morning Weight: __________________

Exercise: __________________

Baby Movements or Activity:

____

Today I am

____

Because _____________________________

____

Blood Sugar Tracking:

AM/Fasting: ________ After Lunch: ________

After Breakfast: ________ After Supper: ________

Enjoyable Exercises: Pelvic Tilts

Pelvic tilts are a great exercise to strengthen abdominal muscles while relieving low back pain. Kneel on your hands and knees with a flat back and without letting your lower back sag toward the floor. Tighten your abdominal muscles, tuck your pelvis, and round your lower back. Hold the pose for several seconds, and release. Continue to round and release rhythmically. Consider asking your partner for a back rub when you're done with the stretching, which will relax you even more. Some experts think being on all fours will get baby into an optimal position for the birth. In labor, pelvic tilts can be done to help a baby rotate and move down in the birth canal.

Morning	Carbs	Lunch	Carbs	Supper	Carbs	Snacks	Carbs

Medications taken today:

Today I am 29 Weeks and 5 Days Pregnant

Date: ____________________________ Day of Week: Su M T W Th F Sa

Morning Weight: ________________

Exercise: ________________

Baby Movements or Activity:

____

Today I am

____

Because ______________________________

____

Blood Sugar Tracking:

AM/Fasting: ________ After Lunch: ________

After Breakfast: ________ After Supper: ________

Questions To Ask Your Doctor

Part of the anxiety about birth – especially if this is your first baby – is not knowing exactly what will happen. You can begin to prepare by learning more about your healthcare provider's and birth location's typical routines. Find out who you can have with your for the birth, and what the typical procedures are when you are admitted in labor. Ask if you can walk or move as needed to find comfort during labor. Ask the doctor what circumstances will lead to interventions, and what will happen if complications arise. Find out how your baby will be cared for after a normal birth and if problems occur. A little knowledge goes a long way to make you less fearful going into childbirth.

Morning	Carbs	Lunch	Carbs	Supper	Carbs	Snacks	Carbs

Medications taken today:

Today I am 29 Weeks and 6 Days Pregnant

Date: ______________________________ Day of Week: Su M T W Th F Sa

Morning Weight: ______________

Exercise: ______________________

Baby Movements or Activity:

____

Today I am

____

Because ______________________

____

Blood Sugar Tracking:

AM/Fasting: ________ After Lunch: ________

After Breakfast: ________ After Supper: ________

Tips For Traveling When Pregnant

If you don't have any complications, travel during pregnancy is typically fine. The best place to start your planning is to ask your healthcare provider if you have any risk factors that would limit your ability to travel. Let your provider know if you plan to travel by land or by air, as this may make a difference in his or her recommendations. Dress comfortably for the event, wearing loose clothing, including socks and shoes. Make sure you are stretching as often as possible, and use the restroom as soon as you feel the urge. If you are traveling by car, always wear your seatbelt. Seat belts do not increase the risk of injury to you or your baby, but actually protect you both. Wear the lap portion across your hips and under your belly, and the shoulder portion across your chest.

Morning	Carbs	Lunch	Carbs	Supper	Carbs	Snacks	Carbs

Medications taken today:

Today I am 29 Weeks and 7 Days Pregnant

Date: ______________________________ Day of Week: Su M T W Th F Sa

Morning Weight: __________________

Exercise: _______________________

Baby Movements or Activity:

____

Today I am

____

Because _____________________________

____

Blood Sugar Tracking:

AM/Fasting: _________ After Lunch: _________

After Breakfast: _________ After Supper: _________

Learn About Newborn Care

Many new parents have never cared for a newborn baby. Some have never held a little one. No matter how much experience you have, learning about newborn care can ease the transition from pregnancy to parenthood. Consider taking a class to learn to feed, bathe and diaper your baby. These courses often include information about when to call the doctor, as well as what is normal for newborns. Visit friends or family with a little baby. Ask questions about what their biggest newborn challenges have been. Read as much as you can about growth and development. Taking these steps will help you feel confident in caring for your new family member.

Morning	Carbs	Lunch	Carbs	Supper	Carbs	Snacks	Carbs

Medications taken today:

Overview Of My 29th Week:

Doctor's Visits Notes:

A Picture To Remember This Week

Today I am 30 Weeks and 1 Day Pregnant

Date: ______________________________ Day of Week: Su M T W Th F Sa

Morning Weight: __________________

Exercise: __________________

Baby Movements or Activity:

____

Today I am

____

Because ____________________________

____

Blood Sugar Tracking:

AM/Fasting: ________ After Lunch: ________

After Breakfast: ________ After Supper: ________

Nutrition Nugget: Don't Skip Breakfast

Many of us have heard that breakfast is the most important meal of the day; but, with our busy lives, eating early sometimes gets overlooked. Pregnancy is no time to skip this essential meal. Eating breakfast sets your metabolism for the entire day, making you less prone to binge snacking or giving in to cravings later in the afternoon. Breakfast provides you with energy – and gets your baby a steady supply of nutrients after the overnight period. If you are experiencing morning sickness, eating a few bites before getting out of bed may help. Some researchers have even linked skipping breakfast with preterm labor. Why take the risk?

Morning	Carbs	Lunch	Carbs	Supper	Carbs	Snacks	Carbs

Medications taken today:

Today I am 30 Weeks and 2 Days Pregnant

Date: ____________________________ Day of Week: Su M T W Th F Sa

Morning Weight: ________________

Exercise: ______________________

Baby Movements or Activity:

____

Today I am

____

Because ________________________

____

Blood Sugar Tracking:

AM/Fasting: ________ After Lunch: ________

After Breakfast: ________ After Supper: ________

Keeping Yourself Comfortable: Heartburn

As your third trimester progresses, you may be more prone to suffer from heartburn. Caused by hormonal changes, heartburn happens when the valve separating the esophagus from the stomach doesn't fully close and allows stomach acids to move back up. Dietary changes to prevent or treat heartburn include eating small meals, drinking between rather than with meals, avoiding spicy and fatty foods, and avoiding carbonated beverages. You may need to sleep propped up, and keep from laying down right after eating. What sounds like an old wives' tale - if you have heartburn, your baby will be born with lots of hair - is strangely true. More than 80% of women who have heartburn give birth to babies with lots of hair.

Morning	Carbs	Lunch	Carbs	Supper	Carbs	Snacks	Carbs

Medications taken today:

Today I am 30 Weeks and 3 Days Pregnant

Date: ______________________________ Day of Week: Su M T W Th F Sa

Morning Weight: __________________

Exercise: _______________________

Baby Movements or Activity:

____

Today I am

____

Because ___________________________

____

Blood Sugar Tracking:

AM/Fasting: _________ After Lunch: _________

After Breakfast: _________ After Supper: _________

Oh Baby!

About the size of a cantaloupe, your baby now weighs about 3 pounds and is almost 16 inches from head to heel. A pint and a half of amniotic fluid surrounds your baby, and that amount will naturally decrease as he takes up more room in the womb. Brain development still takes center stage - this week, the brain begins to take on its wrinkled appearance as folds, called gyri, make room for more brain cells. Red blood cells are now forming in your baby's bone marrow, too. Lanugo, the downy hair covering and protecting your baby's skin, starts to disappear, though he may still have some after birth.

Morning	Carbs	Lunch	Carbs	Supper	Carbs	Snacks	Carbs

Medications taken today:

Today I am 30 Weeks and 4 Days Pregnant

Date: ______________________________ Day of Week: Su M T W Th F Sa

Morning Weight: __________________

Exercise: ___________________

Baby Movements or Activity:

____

Today I am

____

Because ____________________________

____

Blood Sugar Tracking:

AM/Fasting: ________ After Lunch: ________

After Breakfast: ________ After Supper: ________

Kegel Exercises

Kegel exercises are movements to tone your pelvic floor muscles. Having these tissues in shape before birth can help when it comes to delivering your baby. If you imagine a hammock between your pelvic bone and your tailbone, that's where you pelvic floor is located. You can tone this muscle by clenching and releasing it in a variety of ways. Doing Kegels as often as you can remember has many benefits including better muscle tone (which can lead to more efficient pushing in labor), improved circulation (which will help with healing after the birth), decreased incontinence, and enhanced sexual pleasure.

Morning	Carbs	Lunch	Carbs	Supper	Carbs	Snacks	Carbs

Medications taken today:

Today I am 30 Weeks and 5 Days Pregnant

Date: ______________________________ Day of Week: Su M T W Th F Sa

Morning Weight: __________________

Exercise: __________________

Baby Movements or Activity:

____

Today I am

____

Because ______________________________

____

Blood Sugar Tracking:

AM/Fasting: ________ After Lunch: ________

After Breakfast: ________ After Supper: ________

Hormones Cocktail: Oxytocin

Oxytocin is the hormone of love and altruism. It's highest during pregnancy, birth and breastfeeding, as well as during orgasm. Our bodies even release oxytocin when we share a meal with friends. During pregnancy, oxytocin enhances nutrient absorption, reduces stress, and conserves energy. During the birth process, oxytocin causes the uterine contractions as well as the "fetal ejection reflex," that final surge the woman's body gives when the baby's head is about to be born. It continues to be released to aid the delivery of the placenta. In breastfeeding, oxytocin stimulates the "let-down" reflex. Researchers have even found that mothers who breastfed for more than seven weeks were calmer when their babies were six months old than mothers who did not breastfeed at all.

Morning	Carbs	Lunch	Carbs	Supper	Carbs	Snacks	Carbs

Medications taken today:

Today I am 30 Weeks and 6 Days Pregnant

Date: ______________________________ Day of Week: Su M T W Th F Sa

Morning Weight: ________________

Exercise: ______________________

Baby Movements or Activity:

____

Today I am

____

Because _________________________

____

Blood Sugar Tracking:

AM/Fasting: ________ After Lunch: ________

After Breakfast: ________ After Supper: ________

Choosing the Right Bra for Pregnancy and Breastfeeding

Over the course of your pregnancy, you have probably noticed many breast changes, including a darker areola, more prominent nipples, and more noticeable veins. But the biggest alteration may be in breast size! Now is the time to shop for a comfortable maternity bra, or consider buying some nursing bras. It's best to be professionally fitted, since your cup and band size are likely different than normal, and you should probably purchase several. Be sure the new lingerie is well constructed and supportive, and made of a breathable fabric. Some experts recommend not buying underwire bras, as they can cause plugged ducts, though many companies now make soft-wire support that is safer for nursing moms.

Morning	Carbs	Lunch	Carbs	Supper	Carbs	Snacks	Carbs

Medications taken today:

Today I am 30 Weeks and 7 Days Pregnant

Date: ______________________________ Day of Week: Su M T W Th F Sa

Morning Weight: ________________

Exercise: ________________

Baby Movements or Activity:

____

Today I am

____

Because ______________________________

____

Blood Sugar Tracking:

AM/Fasting: _________ After Lunch: _________

After Breakfast: _________ After Supper: _________

Pregnancy Traditions: Food Taboos

Cultures around the world have restrictions on what pregnant moms should eat. In some African countries, mothers are told not to eat eggs, milk and meat, because it will increase libido, and sex is thought harm the growing baby. In Sri Lanka, mothers are warned against mangoes, vinegar, and pineapple, which are thought to cause miscarriage. Traditionally, Japanese women were not allowed to eat any seafood with claws (such as crabs or lobsters) so the child wouldn't become a thief. They were also discouraged from eating squid or persimmons, which could make the uterus "cold" and lead to miscarriage.

Morning	Carbs	Lunch	Carbs	Supper	Carbs	Snacks	Carbs

Medications taken today:

Overview Of My 30th Week:

Doctor's Visits Notes:

A Picture To Remember This Week

Today I am 31 Weeks and 1 Day Pregnant

Date: ______________________________ Day of Week: Su M T W Th F Sa

Morning Weight: __________________

Exercise: _______________________

Baby Movements or Activity:

____

Today I am

____

Because ___________________________

____

Blood Sugar Tracking:

AM/Fasting: ________ After Lunch: __________

After Breakfast: _________ After Supper: _________

Nutrition Nugget: Good Fats

Essential fatty acids (EFAs), like Omega-3 and Omega-6, are a necessity for brain growth before and after birth. These EFAs also optimize baby's retinal development. Experts recommend 300–600 mg of DHA (an essential fatty acid) each day during pregnancy and breastfeeding. EFAs most easily processed by the body can be found in oily fish (such as herring, sardines, and salmon) and in fish-oil supplements. If you have an aversion or allergy to fish and can't take fish-oil supplements, there are plant-based sources of EFAs; however, these plant-based sources aren't as easy for the body to process. The best plant-based sources of EFAs are flaxseed oil, canola oil, chia seeds, walnuts, walnut oil, grass-reared meat, and dark green leafy vegetables, such as spinach and kale.

Morning	Carbs	Lunch	Carbs	Supper	Carbs	Snacks	Carbs

Medications taken today:

Today I am 31 Weeks and 2 Days Pregnant

Date: ______________________________ Day of Week: Su M T W Th F Sa

Morning Weight: ________________

Exercise: ____________________

Baby Movements or Activity:

____

Today I am

____

Because ______________________________

____

Blood Sugar Tracking:

AM/Fasting: ________ After Lunch: ________

After Breakfast: ________ After Supper: ________

Coping with Mood Swings

Mood swings are a normal part of pregnancy – for both men and women. One minute you're feeling excitement and joy, and the next you are apprehensive and anxious about pregnancy, labor, birth, and parenting. All parents-to-be go through these changes. While you have hormones partially to blame, the huge life change that a new baby brings is hard on both partners. If mood swings are impacting your relationship, talk to each other about what's bothering you. Chances are you are sharing the same fears. One of the best ways to counteract mood swings is to increase endorphins, nature's narcotic, though exercise.

Morning	Carbs	Lunch	Carbs	Supper	Carbs	Snacks	Carbs

Medications taken today:

Today I am 31 Weeks and 3 Days Pregnant

Date: ______________________________ Day of Week: Su M T W Th F Sa

Morning Weight: ____________________

Exercise: ________________________

Baby Movements or Activity:

____

Today I am

____

Because ___________________________

____

Blood Sugar Tracking:

AM/Fasting: ________ After Lunch: __________

After Breakfast: __________ After Supper: __________

Oh Baby!

Your baby may weigh as much as a gallon of milk and will double in weight between this week and birth. The bones are beginning to harden, which means your baby's calcium needs are increased. While he is likely still pretty active, don't worry if it seems like there are fewer movements as the weeks progress. Your baby's movements are simply becoming less erratic and more organized due to the maturation of the nervous system. The brain is developed to the point where he can process information, track light and perceive all five senses. Sleep stretches are longer now, too, accounting for the stillness. Not to mention that there's just not as much room in the uterus anymore! Keep a kick count if you're worried – lie down and count for one hour. As long as you feel at least 10 kicks, your baby is doing fine.

Morning	Carbs	Lunch	Carbs	Supper	Carbs	Snacks	Carbs

Medications taken today:

Today I am 31 Weeks and 4 Days Pregnant

Date: ______________________________ Day of Week: Su M T W Th F Sa

Morning Weight: __________________

Exercise: ________________________

Baby Movements or Activity:

____

Today I am

____

Because ___________________________

____

Blood Sugar Tracking:

AM/Fasting: ________ After Lunch: ________

After Breakfast: ________ After Supper: ________

What's So Great About Relaxation?

Relaxation is best defined as the art of releasing muscle tension. Childbirth experts have found that women who cope well with labor without using pain medications all exhibit three common traits: they have a ritual to get through contractions, they use rhythm to manage each contraction, and they use active relaxation techniques for comfort. While the rhythm and ritual are typically spontaneous, relaxation can be learned beforehand. The benefits of relaxation extend beyond pregnancy and birth, and include: peace and a sense of well-being, improved posture, reduced stress, energy conservation, reduced fatigue, and increased oxygenation. This last benefit is important when it comes to the uterine and pelvic muscles and to the fetus during labor!

Morning	Carbs	Lunch	Carbs	Supper	Carbs	Snacks	Carbs

Medications taken today:

Today I am 31 Weeks and 5 Days Pregnant

Date: ______________________________ Day of Week: Su M T W Th F Sa

Morning Weight: __________________

Exercise: ____________________

Baby Movements or Activity:

____

Today I am

____

Because ______________________________

____

Blood Sugar Tracking:

AM/Fasting: ________ After Lunch: ________

After Breakfast: ________ After Supper: ________

Hormones Cocktail: Cathecholamines

The cathecholamines are the fight-or-flight hormones, adrenaline and nor-adrenaline. They are released in response to anxiety, fright, hunger and cold, as well as excitement. They prepare the body to get away from danger by reducing blood flow to non-essential organs and sending it instead to those most needed for escape. High levels of catecholamines have been associated with longer labor and changes to the fetal heart rate. Animals in the wild, when started, will stop labor until they feel safe again. Humans are no different. The best way to limit the adrenaline interference with labor is to create a space where you feel safe to let your body do the work of birth.

Morning	Carbs	Lunch	Carbs	Supper	Carbs	Snacks	Carbs

Medications taken today:

Today I am 31 Weeks and 6 Days Pregnant

Date: ______________________________ Day of Week: Su M T W Th F Sa

Morning Weight: __________________

Exercise: ________________________

Baby Movements or Activity:

____

Today I am

____

Because __________________________

____

Blood Sugar Tracking:

AM/Fasting: _________ After Lunch: _________

After Breakfast: _________ After Supper: _________

Dealing with stress in pregnancy

Knowing your stressors is the first step in dealing with them. You could be worrying about birth or your baby's health, or maybe financial issues or family dynamics are causing you to feel anxious. Creating a stress management plan is a life skill that you can work on now during pregnancy.. Start by considering what all of your joys and fears are for this pregnancy – write them down if you need to. Then consider which ones you have control over, and which are out of your power to change. Come up with ways to deal with each individual fear before birth. If situations not related to pregnancy are causing issues, what can you do to change them? Dealing now with life stressors will benefit you and your new baby as you move into the next phase of your life.

Morning	Carbs	Lunch	Carbs	Supper	Carbs	Snacks	Carbs

Medications taken today:

Today I am 31 Weeks and 7 Days Pregnant

Date: ______________________________ Day of Week: Su M T W Th F Sa

Morning Weight: ____________________

Exercise: ____________________

Baby Movements or Activity:

____

Today I am

____

Because ______________________________

____

Blood Sugar Tracking:

AM/Fasting: ________ After Lunch: ________

After Breakfast: ________ After Supper: ________

Pregnancy Traditions: Henna Body Art

Looking for a way to celebrate your growing baby bump? Henna body art is an age-old tradition to honor significant life changes for women, such as marriage, pregnancy and childbirth. Practiced for over 5000 years in Middle Eastern, African countries and India, henna body art (sometimes called mehndi) uses a paste created from the dried and ground leaves of the henna plant to stain and cool the skin. Traditionally, henna art in pregnancy was a token to bless and protect the growing child. If you want to try henna, start with a small patch test to be sure you're not allergic. Choose a kit specifically for pregnant moms with all-natural ingredients. Ask your healthcare provider if you have any contraindications that would limit your henna use, such as anemia or jaundice.

Morning	Carbs	Lunch	Carbs	Supper	Carbs	Snacks	Carbs

Medications taken today:

Overview Of My 31st Week:

Doctor's Visits Notes:

A Picture To Remember This Week

Today I am 32 Weeks and 1 Day Pregnant

Date: ______________________________ Day of Week: Su M T W Th F Sa

Morning Weight: ____________________

Exercise: ________________________

Baby Movements or Activity:

____

Today I am

____

Because ______________________________

____

Blood Sugar Tracking:

AM/Fasting: ________ After Lunch: ________

After Breakfast: ________ After Supper: ________

Nutrition Nugget: Smart Snacking

You're always hungry during pregnancy – that's only natural as you're growing another human being. But overeating can lead to complications like excessive weight gain, high blood pressure and gestational diabetes. Smart snacking is the key to keeping you feeling fuller longer and maintaining a stable blood sugar level. Snacks should be small and nutrient dense, and should be spread out between meals. Make sure you are eating because you're actually hungry, and not because you're lonely or anxious. If you find yourself using food for stress relief, see if you can replace those snacks with more healthy alternatives like exercising or talking to a trusted friend.

Morning	Carbs	Lunch	Carbs	Supper	Carbs	Snacks	Carbs

Medications taken today:

Today I am 32 Weeks and 2 Days Pregnant

Date: ______________________________ Day of Week: Su M T W Th F Sa

Morning Weight: ______________________

Exercise: ______________________

Baby Movements or Activity:

____

Today I am

____

Because _______________________________________

____

Blood Sugar Tracking:

AM/Fasting: _________ After Lunch: _________

After Breakfast: _________ After Supper: _________

Keeping Yourself Comfortable: Leg Cramps

You're suddenly awakened in the middle of the night with a terrible pain in your leg! Leg cramps are a fairly common occurrence in late pregnancy. Regular exercise and staying hydrated may prevent them. If you are in the midst of a spasm, start stretching your calf by circling your ankle. Some women even ask their partner to help with this by holding the heel and pushing the ball of the foot toward her body. A warm compress and massage can help loosen the cramped muscle. If you get leg cramps regularly, talk to your doctor or a nutritionist about adjusting your calcium / phosphorus ratio. If you have any swelling, redness, tenderness, or warmth in the legs, talk to your doctor right away as these may signal a blood clot.

Morning	Carbs	Lunch	Carbs	Supper	Carbs	Snacks	Carbs

Medications taken today:

Today I am 32 Weeks and 3 Days Pregnant

Date: ___________________________________ Day of Week: Su M T W Th F Sa

Morning Weight: _____________________

Exercise: _________________________

Baby Movements or Activity:

____

Today I am

____

Because ________________________________

____

Blood Sugar Tracking:

AM/Fasting: _________ After Lunch: _________

After Breakfast: _________After Supper: _________

Oh Baby!

By now, your baby weighs about as much as a 4 large oranges – almost 4 pounds – and is around 16.5 inches long when stretched out. But he is all curled up for a while longer. Most babies move into a head-down, or vertex, position by this week. Typically gravity keeps the head low once it's down, since it's baby's heaviest part. Some babies don't turn until the last minute, though, and some keep doing somersaults for a while longer. He is running out of space to get comfortable, so don't be surprised if you end up with a foot or elbow in the ribs. You will be gaining about a pound a week now, and half of that goes directly to your baby's growth.

Morning	Carbs	Lunch	Carbs	Supper	Carbs	Snacks	Carbs

Medications taken today:

Today I am 32 Weeks and 4 Days Pregnant

Date: ______________________________ Day of Week: Su M T W Th F Sa

Morning Weight: __________________

Exercise: __________________

Baby Movements or Activity:

____

Today I am

____

Because __________________________

____

Blood Sugar Tracking:

AM/Fasting: ________ After Lunch: ________

After Breakfast: ________ After Supper: ________

Relaxation Quickie – Breathing Awareness

Breathing can be used to distract you from the discomforts of labor. The first step is becoming aware of how you breathe. When you are falling asleep, pay attention to your breathing. If you can mimic that type of breathing in an everyday stressful situation, you'll have a good start toward mastery. If you stub your toe or bump your elbow, pay attention to how your breathing changes. Learn to change your breathing consciously. Try this exercise: Place your hands on your abdomen, and imagine your breath moving down to that level. Breathe deeply for a while, relaxing with each exhale. Then move your hands to your chest. This more shallow breathing can help you get past the peak of the worst contractions, or past the pain of a stubbed toe.

Morning	Carbs	Lunch	Carbs	Supper	Carbs	Snacks	Carbs

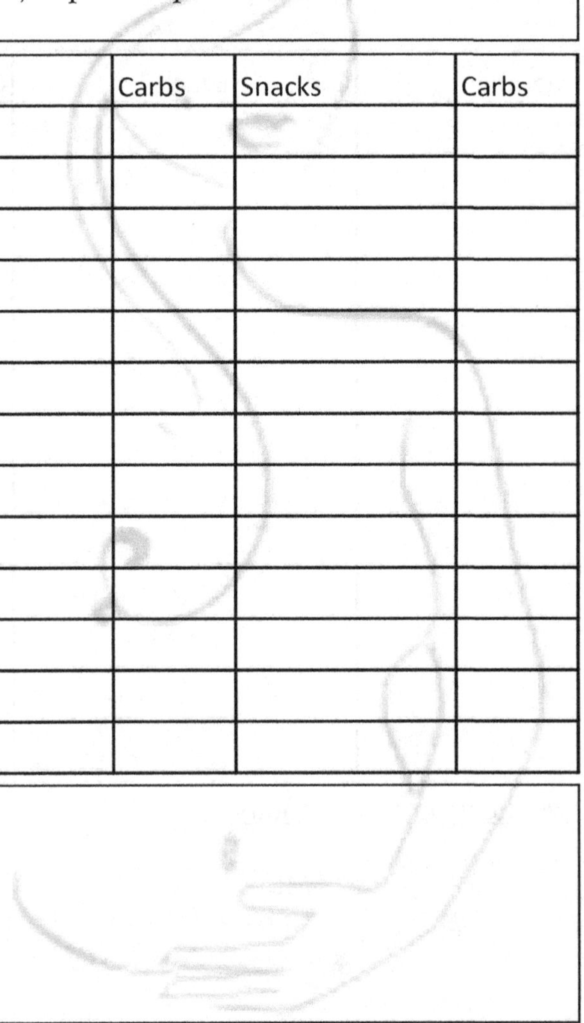

Medications taken today:

Today I am 32 Weeks and 5 Days Pregnant

Date: ______________________________ Day of Week: Su M T W Th F Sa

Morning Weight: ____________________

Exercise: ____________________

Baby Movements or Activity:

____

Today I am

____

Because ______________________________

____

Blood Sugar Tracking:

AM/Fasting: ________ After Lunch: ________

After Breakfast: ________ After Supper: ________

Hormones Cocktail: Endorphins

In response to pain, the body releases natural analgesic substances, called endorphins. High levels of endorphins are present during sex, pregnancy, birth, and breastfeeding. Researchers have found that endorphins start to be release shorty before labor begins. During the birth process, your endorphin levels rise as your contractions increase in intensity, helping you to naturally manage your labor. Endorphins create feelings of mutual dependency – which is one reason women need so much support during childbirth, but is also at the root of mother baby attachment after birth. Pain medications in labor can affect not only mom's endorphin levels, but her baby's as well, and the effects are not well understood.

Morning	Carbs	Lunch	Carbs	Supper	Carbs	Snacks	Carbs

<u>Medications taken today:</u>

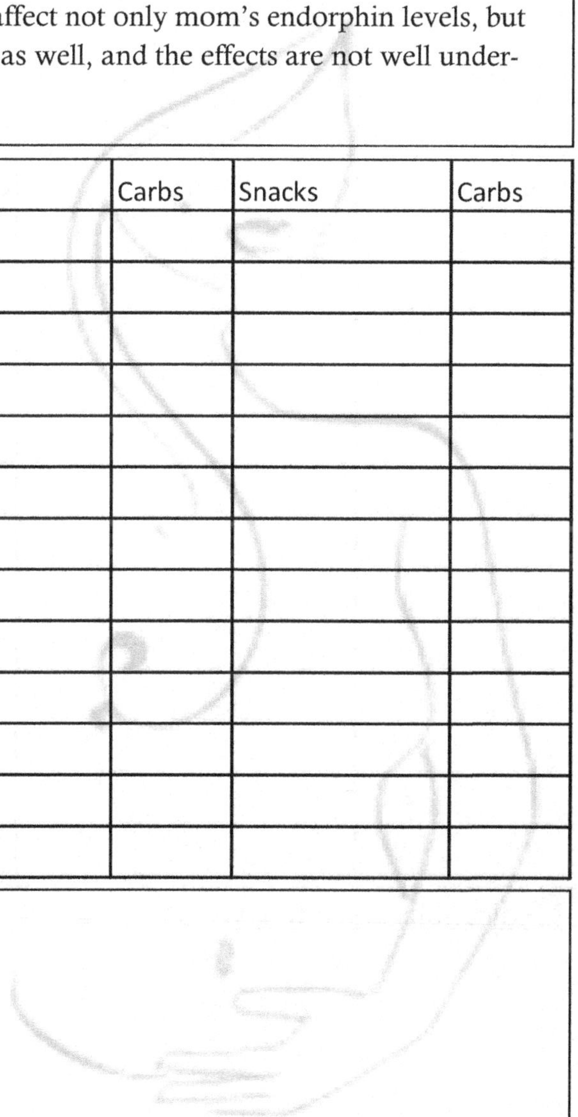

Today I am 32 Weeks and 6 Days Pregnant

Date: ______________________ Day of Week: Su M T W Th F Sa

Morning Weight: ______________

Exercise: ______________________

Baby Movements or Activity:

____

Today I am

____

Because ______________________

____

Blood Sugar Tracking:

AM/Fasting: ________ After Lunch: ________

After Breakfast: ________ After Supper: ________

Sorting Out Pregnancy Symptoms

With all of the strange changes to your body, it's sometimes hard to tell what's normal for pregnancy, and what's something that should be checked by your healthcare provider. Some normal changes of pregnancy that may be bothersome but not medically dangerous include: frequent urination, leg cramps, fatigue, hemorrhoids and varicose veins, heartburn, nausea, stretch marks, nasal congestion – the increased blood volume and fluid retention of pregnancy can cause some congestion, backache, swelling, and breast tenderness. Abnormal changes include progressing contractions before 37 completed weeks, a gush or trickle of fluid from the vagina, local pain or swelling in the legs, fever, sudden weight gain, vaginal bleeding, cramps, burning with urination, and decreased fetal movement. Trust your intuition. If something doesn't feel right, get it checked out.

Morning	Carbs	Lunch	Carbs	Supper	Carbs	Snacks	Carbs

Medications taken today:

Today I am 32 Weeks and 7 Days Pregnant

Date: ______________________________ Day of Week: Su M T W Th F Sa

Morning Weight: __________________

Exercise: __________________

Baby Movements or Activity:

____

Today I am

____

Because ______________________________

____

Blood Sugar Tracking:

AM/Fasting: ________ After Lunch: __________

After Breakfast: ________ After Supper: __________

Read Inspirational Birth Stories

Reading other women's positive birth experiences can encourage you as you move through the discomforts of late pregnancy, and into planning for childbirth. For some reason, people like to share with pregnant moms every birth horror story they've ever heard. Try to push these to the back of your mind, and search for stories that affirm your strength and power as a woman. Look for books or even blogs written from an upbeat, constructive viewpoint. These tales will help you view birth as a natural, safe event, rather than a time fraught with emergencies and negativity. Having a more optimistic outlook can keep you from experiencing a labor stalled by fear later on.

Morning	Carbs	Lunch	Carbs	Supper	Carbs	Snacks	Carbs

<u>Medications taken today:</u>

Overview Of My 32nd Week:

Doctor's Visits Notes:

A Picture To Remember This Week

Today I am 33 Weeks and 1 Day Pregnant

Date: ______________________________ Day of Week: Su M T W Th F Sa

Morning Weight: __________________

Exercise: _______________________

Baby Movements or Activity:

____

Today I am

____

Because ___________________________

____

Blood Sugar Tracking:

AM/Fasting: ________ After Lunch: ________

After Breakfast: ________ After Supper: ________

Nutrition Nugget: Calcium

We've all heard calcium is necessary for strong bones and teeth, and this need is actually increased during pregnancy. Without enough calcium, your baby would have to absorb calcium from you, which can cause your body to suffer. Aside from taking a calcium supplement or being sure your prenatal vitamin contains enough, dietary changes can help. Consider adding more dairy products, such as yogurt or cottage cheese, to your daily diet. Choose low fat or fat free products when you can. Other good sources of calcium include dark salad greens (like spinach), cabbage, broccoli, cucumber, peas, soy, squash, beans (including cocoa), figs, kiwi, almonds, and tomatoes.

Morning	Carbs	Lunch	Carbs	Supper	Carbs	Snacks	Carbs

Medications taken today:

Today I am 33 Weeks and 2 Days Pregnant

Date: ______________________________ Day of Week: Su M T W Th F Sa

Morning Weight: ____________________

Exercise: ________________________

Baby Movements or Activity:

____

Today I am

____

Because ____________________________

____

Be A Goddess

Many cultures around the world and across the ages have woman-centered creation myths. These might be stories of a goddess birthing a culture, or tales about how the world itself was created. Often pregnancy and birth themselves have the protection of a goddess. Creation myths and earth mothers are a way for cultures to explain the unknown. But they can also be a way for modern mothers to feel more connected with creation. Now that you are pregnant, you are a goddess! Allow yourself to feel that kinship with other women now and in the past. Feel connected to creation. Know you are part of the cycle of life, no matter what culture or religion you belong to.

Blood Sugar Tracking:

AM/Fasting: _________ After Lunch: __________

After Breakfast: __________ After Supper: __________

Morning	Carbs	Lunch	Carbs	Supper	Carbs	Snacks	Carbs

Medications taken today:

Today I am 33 Weeks and 3 Days Pregnant

Date: ______________________________ Day of Week: Su M T W Th F Sa

Morning Weight: ____________________

Exercise: ____________________

Baby Movements or Activity:

____

Today I am

____

Because ____________________________

____

Oh Baby!

Now about the size of a pineapple, your baby weighs a little over 4 pounds and has passed the 17-inch mark. Your baby's head circumference has increased by nearly half an inch just this week from the tremendous amount of brain growth. He will grow another full inch in length this week, too. All this growth requires additional protein and fat, and this need will continue over the next few weeks. The level of amniotic fluid level has reached its maximum, and will stay the same until the end of pregnancy. There's plenty to continue protecting your baby. Your baby's skeleton is hardening. The bones in his skull, however, aren't fused together, which makes birthing easier since the bones can overlap to fit better through the birth canal.

Blood Sugar Tracking:

AM/Fasting: ________ After Lunch: ________

After Breakfast: ________ After Supper: ________

Morning	Carbs	Lunch	Carbs	Supper	Carbs	Snacks	Carbs

Medications taken today:

Today I am 33 Weeks and 4 Days Pregnant

Date: ______________________________ Day of Week: Su M T W Th F Sa

Morning Weight: __________________

Exercise: _______________________

Baby Movements or Activity:

____

Today I am

____

Because __________________________

____

Blood Sugar Tracking:

AM/Fasting: ________ After Lunch: ________

After Breakfast: ________ After Supper: ________

Relaxation Quickie: Massage

Try this easy hand massage with your partner's help: let him hold your hand in a well-supported position and start squeezing gently to loosen the muscles. Then your partner can use his thumbs to make small circles all around the palm. Next, he can massage and pull each finger gently. Turn your hand over, and allow him to stroke your hand firmly from the center out to both sides. Use a natural oil to smooth the movements – apricot, sweet almond, coconut or olive oil all work well. During pregnancy, this can relieve tension and during labor it can be used to help you get through contractions or relax between.

Morning	Carbs	Lunch	Carbs	Supper	Carbs	Snacks	Carbs

Medications taken today:

Today I am 33 Weeks and 5 Days Pregnant

Date: ______________________ Day of Week: Su M T W Th F Sa

Morning Weight: ________________

Exercise: ________________

Baby Movements or Activity:

____

Today I am

____

Because ______________________

____

The Fear-Tension-Pain Cycle

This theory of pain management for childbirth suggests the more fear you have, the greater your muscle tension will be, and the more pain you will feel. By mastering any of the three components, you can control your response to labor. By learning more about the birth process and trusting your body, you will be less fearful. By utilizing massage and active relaxation, you will have less tension. By using other comfort measures you will experience less pain. You have the ability to turn the negative spiral that could stall labor around into a more positive force to help you birth your baby.

Blood Sugar Tracking:

AM/Fasting: ________ After Lunch: ________

After Breakfast: ________ After Supper: ________

Morning	Carbs	Lunch	Carbs	Supper	Carbs	Snacks	Carbs

Medications taken today:

Today I am 33 Weeks and 6 Days Pregnant

Date: ______________________________ Day of Week: Su M T W Th F Sa

Morning Weight: ______________________

Exercise: _______________________

Baby Movements or Activity:

____

Today I am

____

Because ____________________________

____

Blood Sugar Tracking:

AM/Fasting: ________ After Lunch: ________

After Breakfast: ________ After Supper: ________

Rethinking Labor Pain

Most women's fears surrounding labor come from wondering how painful it will be. They've all hear horror stories, or seen movies depicting women in the throes of labor desperate for relief. But thinking about labor pain in a more productive way may help alleviate some of those fears. Labor pain means your body is doing what it should to birth your baby – your uterus is contracting to open for the baby, and the baby is moving through the pelvis then into the birth canal. The great thing about these contractions is that they're intermittent – they ebb and flow as labor progresses and they typically last 60 to 90 seconds. There's always a resting period in between. Plan active techniques for getting through one contraction at a time, and for relaxing in between contractions.

Morning	Carbs	Lunch	Carbs	Supper	Carbs	Snacks	Carbs

Medications taken today:

Today I am 33 Weeks and 7 Days Pregnant

Date: ________________________________ Day of Week: Su M T W Th F Sa

Morning Weight: ____________________

Exercise: ________________________

Baby Movements or Activity:

____

Today I am

____

Because ____________________________

____

Blood Sugar Tracking:

AM/Fasting: _________ After Lunch: _________

After Breakfast: _________ After Supper: _________

The Baby Plan

If you have written a birth plan to prepare for labor, you may want to consider carrying on the planning and writing one for life after baby. Sit down with your partner and talk about who will do what after the baby is born. Are you planning to breastfeed, or will bottles need to be prepared and cleaned? Who will do the cooking and food shopping? How will dishes get done, and the toilet get cleaned? Having a plan in place ahead of time will help as you adjust from being a couple to now being a family with a 24/7 responsibility!

Morning	Carbs	Lunch	Carbs	Supper	Carbs	Snacks	Carbs

Medications taken today:

Overview Of My 33rd Week:

Doctor's Visits Notes:

A Picture To Remember This Week

Today I am 34 Weeks and 1 Day Pregnant

Date: ______________________________ Day of Week: Su M T W Th F Sa

Morning Weight: __________________

Exercise: _______________________

Baby Movements or Activity:

____

Today I am

____

Because ___________________________

____

Blood Sugar Tracking:

AM/Fasting: ________ After Lunch: _________

After Breakfast: _________ After Supper: _________

Nutrition Nugget: Iron

Iron is necessary for carrying oxygen to your baby, as well as preventing low birth weight, preterm labor and anemia. It aids in brain development and supports your immune system. Your need for iron during pregnancy actually doubles because of your expanded blood volume. Most prenatal vitamins contain iron, and if they don't, your doctor may suggest you take an additional supplement. Pregnant women need 27 milligrams of iron per day. Good dietary sources of iron include lean red meat, pork, dark poultry meat, liver, eggs, dried fruits, legumes, dried beans, oatmeal, and whole grains. Iron absorption is improved in conjunction with vitamin C, so consider some oranges, strawberries or broccoli with your iron-rich meal.

Morning	Carbs	Lunch	Carbs	Supper	Carbs	Snacks	Carbs

Medications taken today:

Today I am 34 Weeks and 2 Days Pregnant

Date: ______________________________ Day of Week: Su M T W Th F Sa

Morning Weight: ________________

Exercise: ______________________

Baby Movements or Activity:

____

Today I am

____

Because ________________________

____

Keeping Yourself Comfortable: Shortness of Breath

Your body requires more oxygen during pregnancy, and, in fact, pregnancy hormones cause changes in your lungs and brain to help compensate. As your baby starts to run out of space in your abdomen, your little one pushes into your diaphragm, keeping you from taking a deep breath. As you move closer to your due date and your baby engages in the pelvis, you might get some relief. In the meantime, don't push yourself too hard, and if you feel short of breath slow down or take a break from what you're doing. Make sure you are practicing good posture so your lungs have plenty of room to expand. Sleeping propped on pillows may help. Once baby is born, this problem should disappear.

Blood Sugar Tracking:

AM/Fasting: ________ After Lunch: ________

After Breakfast: ________ After Supper: ________

Morning	Carbs	Lunch	Carbs	Supper	Carbs	Snacks	Carbs

Medications taken today:

Today I am 34 Weeks and 3 Days Pregnant

Date: ______________________________ Day of Week: Su M T W Th F Sa

Morning Weight: __________________

Exercise: _______________________

Baby Movements or Activity:

____

Today I am

____

Because ___________________________

____

Blood Sugar Tracking:

AM/Fasting: _________ After Lunch: __________

After Breakfast: _________ After Supper: __________

Oh Baby!

Your baby now weighs almost as much as a bag of sugar - around 4.75 pounds - and is almost 18 inches long. If your little one is a boy, his testicles are starting to descend into his scrotum. Occasionally boys are born with undescended testicles - it's nothing to worry about, they usually move down on their own during baby's first year. While your baby has relied upon your immune system to keep safe throughout pregnancy, this week the fetal immune system starts kicking into high gear. Vernix, a thick, white coating protecting your baby's skin is getting thicker, and will help baby slide more easily through the birth canal.

Morning	Carbs	Lunch	Carbs	Supper	Carbs	Snacks	Carbs

Medications taken today:

Today I am 34 Weeks and 4 Days Pregnant

Date: ______________________________ Day of Week: Su M T W Th F Sa

Morning Weight: __________________

Exercise: _______________________

Baby Movements or Activity:

____

Today I am

____

Because ___________________________

____

Blood Sugar Tracking:

AM/Fasting: ________ After Lunch: ________

After Breakfast: ________ After Supper: ________

Relaxation Quickie: Phrases from Within

Positive self-talk is a powerful tool – even during labor. Start by thinking about how relaxation feels. Describe it to yourself, writing it down if you need to. Then break your script up into short phrases that you can repeat over and over to yourself. By practicing on a regular basis, you can learn to release tension as you say or hear the phrases. For instance, you might say, "my shoulders are loose and warm" and consciously relax your shoulders at the same time. Other phrases used during labor can be more directly linked to birth, such as "my cervix is opening like the petals of a rose" or "my body is opening wide for my baby."

Morning	Carbs	Lunch	Carbs	Supper	Carbs	Snacks	Carbs

Medications taken today:

Today I am 34 Weeks and 5 Days Pregnant

Date: ______________________________ Day of Week: Su M T W Th F Sa

Morning Weight: __________________

Exercise: ______________________

Baby Movements or Activity:

____

Today I am

____

Because _________________________________

____

Blood Sugar Tracking:

AM/Fasting: _________ After Lunch: _________

After Breakfast: _________ After Supper: _________

Natural Birth vs. Pain Medications

As you get closer to your due date, you are probably thinking more and more about birth. One of the main decisions women make is whether they want a natural birth, or if they think pain medication might be better for them. Consider how you feel about medical interventions in general, since pain meds for labor rarely come without other procedures such as IV fluids, bladder catheters, and more. Learn as much as you can about your options so you can make a truly informed choice. If you want to aim for an unmedicated birth, take a childbirth preparation class and learn as many non-pharmacologic comfort measures as you can.

Morning	Carbs	Lunch	Carbs	Supper	Carbs	Snacks	Carbs

Medications taken today:

Today I am 34 Weeks and 6 Days Pregnant

Date: ______________________________ Day of Week: Su M T W Th F Sa

Morning Weight: __________________

Exercise: ________________________

Baby Movements or Activity:

____

Today I am

____

Because __________________________

____

Blood Sugar Tracking:

AM/Fasting: ________ After Lunch: __________

After Breakfast: __________After Supper: __________

Belly Mapping

Ever wonder what each of those bulges is all around your belly? A process called Belly Mapping can help you figure out your baby's position in the uterus during the final weeks of pregnancy. While you may be able to use this method to identify a baby who is malpositioned, most moms do it just for fun. The round firm area is likely where baby's bottom is located. You can probably feel kicks in only specific areas late in pregnancy – this is where the legs, feet, hands and arms are located. Where your healthcare provider hears the heartbeat is the baby's upper back. Have fun guessing!

Morning	Carbs	Lunch	Carbs	Supper	Carbs	Snacks	Carbs

Medications taken today:

Today I am 34 Weeks and 7 Days Pregnant

Date: ______________________________ Day of Week: Su M T W Th F Sa

Morning Weight: ____________________

Exercise: ____________________

Baby Movements or Activity:

____

Today I am

____

Because ______________________________

____

Blood Sugar Tracking:

AM/Fasting: _________ After Lunch: _________

After Breakfast: _________ After Supper: _________

Nutrition Nugget: Artificial Sweeteners and Sugar-free Foods

Nutritive sweeteners (table sugar, sucrose, dextrose, honey, corn sugar, fructose, and maltose) are considered safe to use during pregnancy as long as they aren't used in excess and are counted in your carbohydrate amounts for your day. Women with gestational diabetes, diabetes mellitus, or insulin resistance, however, need to limit their use of nutritive sweeteners. Non-nutritive sweeteners have a sweetening effect without the added calories. They are used in dietetic or reduced calorie foods and beverages. Research is limited on the safety of the use of non-nutritive sweeteners during pregnancy, though the following are considered safe: stevia, aspartame, and sucralose. Pregnant women should avoid saccharin, which may cause problems for the fetus.

Morning	Carbs	Lunch	Carbs	Supper	Carbs	Snacks	Carbs

Medications taken today:

Overview Of My 34th Week:

Doctor's Visits Notes:

A Picture To Remember This Week

Today I am 35 Weeks and 1 Day Pregnant

Date: ______________________________ Day of Week: Su M T W Th F Sa

Morning Weight: __________________

Exercise: ____________________

Baby Movements or Activity:

____

Today I am

____

Because ______________________________

____

Blood Sugar Tracking:

AM/Fasting: ________ After Lunch: ________

After Breakfast: ________ After Supper: ________

Nutrition Nugget: Vitamin D

Vitamin D supports your immune system, healthy cell division and bone health. It's a necessary component for your body to use calcium and phosphorus, and may be protective against depression. Low levels of vitamin D have been linked to certain types of cancers, autoimmune disease, neurologic disease, insulin resistance, cardiovascular disease, and, in pregnancy, preeclampsia or pregnancy-induced hypertension. Recent studies have found women taking 4,000 IU of vitamin D daily had the greatest benefits in preventing preterm labor and births, as well as infections. The best source of vitamin D is sunlight exposure. Food sources of vitamin D include milk, eggs, beef liver, some fish, and fortified cereals, orange juice, yogurt and margarine.

Morning	Carbs	Lunch	Carbs	Supper	Carbs	Snacks	Carbs

<u>Medications taken today:</u>

Today I am 35 Weeks and 2 Days Pregnant

Date: ______________________________ Day of Week: Su M T W Th F Sa

Morning Weight: __________________

Exercise: _______________________

Baby Movements or Activity:

____

Today I am

____

Because ___________________________

____

Blood Sugar Tracking:

AM/Fasting: ________ After Lunch: ________

After Breakfast: ________ After Supper: ________

Keeping Yourself Comfortable: Varicose Veins

More prominent veins under the skin are a symptom many women notice for the first time during pregnancy. The growing uterus puts pressure on the veins throughout your body, including in your legs, progesterone causes the walls of the blood vessels to relax, and your blood volume is greatly increased during pregnancy. Your legs may feel heavy and achy, especially if you've been standing or walking. Sometimes they itch, throb, or feel like they're burning. While varicose veins are hereditary, try to elevate your legs whenever you can, keep from standing for long periods, and wear support hose - if recommended. A warm bath can sometimes help soothe your tired legs, whether from varicose veins or just from the added weight of pregnancy.

Morning	Carbs	Lunch	Carbs	Supper	Carbs	Snacks	Carbs

Medications taken today:

Today I am 35 Weeks and 3 Days Pregnant

Date: ______________________________ Day of Week: Su M T W Th F Sa

Morning Weight: __________________

Exercise: __________________

Baby Movements or Activity:

____

Today I am

____

Because ______________________________

____

Blood Sugar Tracking:

AM/Fasting: ________ After Lunch: _________

After Breakfast: _________After Supper: _________

Oh Baby!

Your baby now weighs as much as a coconut – around 5.25 pounds – and is almost 19 inches long – which is the average size of a newborn. Even though he won't grow many more inches, he will continue to put on weight. Your baby is starting to lay down 'brown fat' this week, which is designed to help your little one stay warm after delivery. Now that most of your baby's basic development is complete, he is busy practicing everything from sucking and breathing to peeing and smiling. In fact, he's peeing nearly a pint of liquid every day!

Morning	Carbs	Lunch	Carbs	Supper	Carbs	Snacks	Carbs

Medications taken today:

Today I am 35 Weeks and 4 Days Pregnant

Date: ________________________________ Day of Week: Su M T W Th F Sa

Morning Weight: ____________________

Exercise: ____________________

Baby Movements or Activity:

____

Today I am

____

Because ____________________________

____

Blood Sugar Tracking:

AM/Fasting: ________ After Lunch: ________

After Breakfast: ________ After Supper: ________

Relaxation Quickie: Aromatherapy

Your sense of smell is intimately connected with your emotions. You can use this to your advantage in labor by bringing aromatherapy into the birthing room. Essential oils can be mixed with a massage medium, or can be used as a pillow or room spray. Consider lavender for relaxation, or peppermint or citrus for invigoration when you're tired. Other common scents used in labor are clary sage (which relieves tension, brings on labor, and helps with expelling the placenta), jasmine (which dulls uterine pain and strengthens contractions), and neroli (for reducing fear, tension, apprehension, and anxiety).

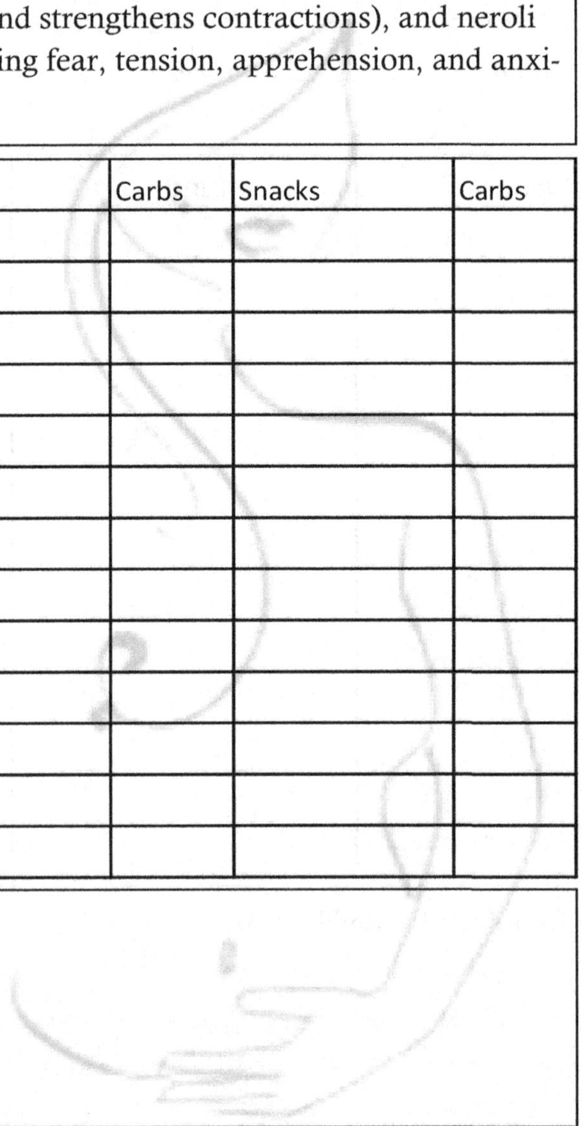

Morning	Carbs	Lunch	Carbs	Supper	Carbs	Snacks	Carbs

Medications taken today:

Today I am 35 Weeks and 5 Days Pregnant

Date: ______________________________ Day of Week: Su M T W Th F Sa

Morning Weight: __________________

Exercise: ____________________

Baby Movements or Activity:

____

Today I am

____

Because ____________________________

____

Must Haves for the Labor Bag

While you've probably packed your nightgown, toiletries and an outfit for the baby, don't forget to pack a bag of tools to support you during labor. You might want some music – relaxing and upbeat – and massagers may help your partner's hands from tiring too soon. If you think massage will be an essential component of your labor, don't forget to pack a natural oil for lubrication. Don't underestimate the effects of aromatherapy. You might need lip balm, candy or gum, too. Consider warm socks or slippers, or a heating pad. Some women find extra pillows useful. And don't forget about your birth partner – he/she may need some snacks to keep up his/her energy!

Blood Sugar Tracking:

AM/Fasting: ________ After Lunch: _________

After Breakfast: _________After Supper: _________

Morning	Carbs	Lunch	Carbs	Supper	Carbs	Snacks	Carbs

Medications taken today:

Today I am 35 Weeks and 6 Days Pregnant

Date: ______________________ Day of Week: Su M T W Th F Sa

Morning Weight: ______________

Exercise: ______________

Baby Movements or Activity:

____

Today I am

____

Because ______________________

____

Blood Sugar Tracking:

AM/Fasting: ________ After Lunch: ________

After Breakfast: ________After Supper: ________

Shut the Gate on Pain

In the 1950s, researchers began to develop the Gate Control Theory of pain management, which suggests you can actively intervene to improve pain management. This theory explains why massage works for pain relief – the touch and pressure sensations of massage get to your brain faster, shutting the gate so that the pain message can't get through. While this theory is most appropriate for labor and birth, you can start to practice now with the normal aches and pains of pregnancy. For example, if your lower back is aching, see if you can gate off the pain with massage of the hands and feet. Or perhaps your partner could try light stroking movements – on your belly or thighs.

Morning	Carbs	Lunch	Carbs	Supper	Carbs	Snacks	Carbs

Medications taken today:

Today I am 35 Weeks and 7 Days Pregnant

Date: ______________________________ Day of Week: Su M T W Th F Sa

Morning Weight: __________________

Exercise: __________________

Baby Movements or Activity:

____

Today I am

____

Because ______________________________

____

Blood Sugar Tracking:

AM/Fasting: ________ After Lunch: ________

After Breakfast: ________ After Supper: ________

Braxton-Hicks Contractions

Occasionally throughout pregnancy, your uterus contracts and releases. Some of these contractions are more noticeable than others, and they are often referred to as Braxton-Hicks or practice contractions. If they happen near the end of pregnancy, you may mistake them for labor, which is how they also earned the name false-labor contractions. These harmless spasms may occur as early as the 6th week of pregnancy. They are typically felt in the abdomen, and can last a minute or two. They tend to happen when you change position, or if you are dehydrated. If you find them especially uncomfortable, practice slow breathing until the spasm passes.

Morning	Carbs	Lunch	Carbs	Supper	Carbs	Snacks	Carbs

Medications taken today:

Overview Of My 35th Week:

Doctor's Visits Notes:

A Picture To Remember This Week

Today I am 36 Weeks and 1 Day Pregnant

Date: ______________________________ Day of Week: Su M T W Th F Sa

Morning Weight: __________________

Exercise: ____________________

Baby Movements or Activity:

____

Today I am

____

Because ______________________________

____

Nutrition Nugget: Vitamin C

Vitamin C is a needed nutrient for tissue repair, wound healing, infection fighting, bone growth and repair, and healthy skin. In pregnancy, it may decrease the risk of miscarriage and pregnancy induced hypertension. It's also helps with iron absorption. Good food sources include citrus fruits and juices (oranges, lemons, limes, grapefruit, etc.), strawberries, tomatoes, red peppers, and broccoli. Some studies show that too much vitamin C may increase the risk of preterm birth, so use caution with additional supplements and consider sticking to only dietary sources. Vitamin C can also cause an upset stomach, so if you are suffering from morning sickness, you may need to steer clear of consuming too much.

Blood Sugar Tracking:

AM/Fasting: _________ After Lunch: __________

After Breakfast: __________ After Supper: __________

Morning	Carbs	Lunch	Carbs	Supper	Carbs	Snacks	Carbs

Medications taken today:

Today I am 36 Weeks and 2 Days Pregnant

Date: ____________________ Day of Week: Su M T W Th F Sa

Morning Weight: ____________________

Exercise: ____________________

Baby Movements or Activity:

____

Today I am

____

Because ____________________

____

Blood Sugar Tracking:

AM/Fasting: __________ After Lunch: __________

After Breakfast: __________ After Supper: __________

Keeping Yourself Comfortable: Hemorrhoids

Hemorrhoids are actually a varicose vein in the rectum. About 20 to 50 percent of pregnant moms develop this uncomfortable condition. Increased blood flow to the pelvis, along with pressure from your growing uterus and an overall slow-down of your digestive system can all contribute. The best way to avoid them is to stay regular by eating enough fiber and staying well hydrated as well as doing Kegel exercises to improve blood flow to the pelvic floor. If you are so unlucky as to have hemorrhoids, you can ease the itch with witch hazel compresses or ice packs. Ask your healthcare provider, though, before using any other treatments.

Morning	Carbs	Lunch	Carbs	Supper	Carbs	Snacks	Carbs

Medications taken today:

Today I am 36 Weeks and 3 Days Pregnant

Date: ______________________ Day of Week: Su M T W Th F Sa

Morning Weight: ______________

Exercise: ______________

Baby Movements or Activity:

____

Today I am

____

Because ______________________

____

Blood Sugar Tracking:

AM/Fasting: ________ After Lunch: ________

After Breakfast: ________ After Supper: ________

Oh Baby!

Your baby is gaining about an ounce a day – tipping the scales at almost 6 pounds and measuring around 20 inches long – about the size of a head of honeydew melon. All this weight gain means baby's calorie demands are still high. Since baby's senses are well developed and he's big enough to be right against the uterine wall, take some time to connect by massaging your belly and talking to your little one. Studies show that newborns prefer their own mother's voice, as well as other sounds commonly heard while in utero. Playing a lullaby over and over now may help with newborn fussiness later!

Morning	Carbs	Lunch	Carbs	Supper	Carbs	Snacks	Carbs

Medications taken today:

Today I am 36 Weeks and 4 Days Pregnant

Date: ______________________________ Day of Week: Su M T W Th F Sa

Morning Weight: __________________

Exercise: __________________

Baby Movements or Activity:

____

Today I am

____

Because ____________________________

____

Blood Sugar Tracking:

AM/Fasting: ________ After Lunch: __________

After Breakfast: _________ After Supper: __________

Relaxation Quickie – Recognizing Tension

In labor, it's important for your partner to be able to tell when – and more importantly where - you're tense. Try this relaxation activity together: tense a part of your body without telling him, and make him figure our where the tension is located. Once he finds your tension, he can use massage to help you relax. Afterwards, return the favor an allow him to tense a muscle for you to find. This not only helps the two of you communicate about your needs, but can be a great way to laugh and unwind after a long day.

Morning	Carbs	Lunch	Carbs	Supper	Carbs	Snacks	Carbs

Medications taken today:

Today I am 36 Weeks and 5 Days Pregnant

Date: ______________________________ Day of Week: Su M T W Th F Sa

Morning Weight: ____________________

Exercise: __________________________

Baby Movements or Activity:

____

Today I am

____

Because _____________________________

____

Blood Sugar Tracking:

AM/Fasting: _________ After Lunch: __________

After Breakfast: __________ After Supper: __________

Hypnosis For Birth?

Hypnosis allows a person to feel completely relaxed, and to block out distractions. During labor, hypnosis can change the pain perception, either through external suggestions during the hypnotized state, or through conditioning before labor starts. This method takes practice, and is best learned from an instructor trained in hypnosis specifically for birth. Classes typically teach women to hypnotize themselves, sometimes with the help of their partner, music, deep breathing, massage, or a verbal script. As women travel into a hypnotic state during labor, partners or support persons can help her see labor in more positive terms, through affirmations or simply more positive word choices (rushes or surges rather than contractions, for instance).

Morning	Carbs	Lunch	Carbs	Supper	Carbs	Snacks	Carbs

Medications taken today:

Today I am 36 Weeks and 6 Days Pregnant

Date: ______________________________ Day of Week: Su M T W Th F Sa

Morning Weight: __________________

Exercise: _______________________

Baby Movements or Activity:

____

Today I am

____

Because _________________________

____

Blood Sugar Tracking:

AM/Fasting: ________ After Lunch: _________

After Breakfast: _________After Supper: _________

Birth Plans

Writing a birth plan can help you sort out all of the options you have for labor, birth and early parenting. It helps you and your partner communicate about your preferences for comfort measures during childbirth, and helps the nursing staff better understand your needs. Your doctor will appreciate knowing more about how you view birth, and can let you know if any of your expectations are unrealistic (Do you want an epidural but still want to walk but your facility doesn't offer that option? Your healthcare provider can spot these discrepancies.) Taking a childbirth preparation class is the best way to learn more about the risks and benefits of all birth options.

Morning	Carbs	Lunch	Carbs	Supper	Carbs	Snacks	Carbs

Medications taken today:

Today I am 36 Weeks and 7 Days Pregnant

Date: ______________________________ Day of Week: Su M T W Th F Sa

Morning Weight: __________________

Exercise: ____________________

Baby Movements or Activity:

____

Today I am

____

Because _____________________________

____

Blood Sugar Tracking:

AM/Fasting: ________ After Lunch: _________

After Breakfast: _________ After Supper: _________

Affirmations for Birth

Positive affirmations are phrases that can help change your mindset about any situation, including pregnancy and birth. Some phrases you might consider repeating to yourself are:

I feel calm and peaceful.

My strong baby is growing big and healthy.

I breathe in energy, and breathe out tension

My body is made to birth this baby.

I am strong and confident.

Affirmations should be present tense, and can be combined with visualization for added effect. Put post-it notes around the house with positive pregnancy thoughts. Or, write some affirmations on index cards, and have your partner read them to you during labor.

Morning	Carbs	Lunch	Carbs	Supper	Carbs	Snacks	Carbs

Medications taken today:

Overview Of My 36th Week:

Doctor's Visits Notes:

A Picture To Remember This Week

Today I am 37 Weeks and 1 Day Pregnant

Date: ________________________________ Day of Week: Su M T W Th F Sa

Morning Weight: ____________________

Exercise: ________________________

Baby Movements or Activity:

____

Today I am

____

Because ______________________________

____

Blood Sugar Tracking:

AM/Fasting: ________ After Lunch: ________

After Breakfast: ________ After Supper: ________

Nutrition Nugget: Fish

Fish is a great source of lean protein and essential fatty acids, building blocks of healthy growth and development. These fatty acids are essential for brain growth – and the third trimester marks leaps and bounds for your baby in that area. But, you may also have heard it's dangerous to eat fish during pregnancy due to high mercury levels in some species. Avoid large fish, such as shark, swordfish, king mackerel, fresh tuna, sea bass, and mahi mahi. If you enjoy canned light tuna, limit consumption to 12 ounces per week. The same is true with shellfish, smaller ocean fish, farm-raised fish, and store-bought freshwater fish. Wild salmon, flounder, haddock, perch, cod, and trout are all considered safe to eat. Just be sure they don't come from contaminated waters.

Morning	Carbs	Lunch	Carbs	Supper	Carbs	Snacks	Carbs

Medications taken today:

Today I am 37 Weeks and 2 Days Pregnant

Date: ______________________________ Day of Week: Su M T W Th F Sa

Morning Weight: ________________

Exercise: ______________________

Baby Movements or Activity:

____

Today I am

____

Because ________________________

____

Blood Sugar Tracking:

AM/Fasting: ________ After Lunch: ________

After Breakfast: ________ After Supper: ________

Preterm Labor: Know the Signs

Since being born too early can lead to many problems for you and your baby, learning to recognize the signs of preterm labor is especially important. If you have four to five contractions in one hour, abdominal cramping, pressure low in the pelvis, a change in vaginal discharge, bleeding, or leaking fluid from the vagina, call your healthcare provider right away. If caught early enough, your doctor may be able to stop your labor from progressing, giving your baby more time to grow and mature before birth. If you think labor might be starting lie down on you left side, and drink lots of water. Keep track of contractions, and if they don't slow, call you doctor or midwife.

Morning	Carbs	Lunch	Carbs	Supper	Carbs	Snacks	Carbs

Medications taken today:

Today I am 37 Weeks and 3 Days Pregnant

Date: ______________________________ Day of Week: Su M T W Th F Sa

Morning Weight: __________________

Exercise: ________________________

Baby Movements or Activity:

____

Today I am

____

Because ___________________________

____

Blood Sugar Tracking:

AM/Fasting: _________ After Lunch: _________

After Breakfast: _________ After Supper: _________

Oh Baby!

You've made it – at the end of this week, you're considered full term. Your baby is the size of a watermelon - around 19 to 20 inches long and weighing between 6 and 6.5 pounds. He'll still be gaining about a half pound a week until birth, putting on fat to keep him warm and help him maintain his blood sugar. Your baby may "drop" this week – don't worry, it just means he might be descending into your pelvis. He should be in a head-down position by now. If not, your care provider may have some suggestions for getting him to turn. Breech presentation at birth – when the his bottom is closest to the birth canal – is more dangerous for both mom and baby, so it's worth the effort to try and get him into a head down position.

Morning	Carbs	Lunch	Carbs	Supper	Carbs	Snacks	Carbs

Medications taken today:

Today I am 37 Weeks and 4 Days Pregnant

Date: ______________________ Day of Week: Su M T W Th F Sa

Morning Weight: ______________________

Exercise: ______________________

Baby Movements or Activity:

____

Today I am

____

Because ______________________

____

Blood Sugar Tracking:

AM/Fasting: ________ After Lunch: ________

After Breakfast: ________ After Supper: ________

Relaxation Quickie – Progressive Relaxation

Progressive relaxation is tensing as well as stretching muscles so that you can find the most relaxed point in between. Start with your face and head, and work your way down your body. For instance, contract your forehead as if you're angry, and release. Then raise your eyebrows in surprise, and release as if someone is smoothing your brow. Can you feel the neutral relaxed point in between? Practicing this method often can condition you to simply get into a well-supported position and let go of overall tension in your body. Find a script and have your partner read it to you in order to practice. Any technique you get good at during pregnancy will come more naturally during labor and birth.

Morning	Carbs	Lunch	Carbs	Supper	Carbs	Snacks	Carbs

Medications taken today:

Today I am 37 Weeks and 5 Days Pregnant

Date: ______________________________ Day of Week: Su M T W Th F Sa

Morning Weight: __________________

Exercise: __________________

Baby Movements or Activity:

____

Today I am

____

Because __________________________

____

Blood Sugar Tracking:

AM/Fasting: ________ After Lunch: ________

After Breakfast: ________ After Supper: ________

How Will I Know I'm in Labor?

A huge gush of water and rushing to the hospital – is this how you imagine the start of labor? In fact, a woman's water breaks at the onset of labor only about 10 percent of the time. What about the other 90 percent? Thankfully, your body will give you signals. The number one positive sign of labor is contractions that get progressively longer, stronger and closer together. Other signs in the last few weeks of pregnancy that let you know labor may be nearing include flu-like symptoms (without a fever), increased backache, increased whitish vaginal discharge, bloody show, lightening (or engagement of the baby in the pelvis), and an increase in the frequency of Braxton-Hicks contractions. It may sound like an old wives' tale, but if you find yourself nesting, it could be a sign that labor is imminent.

Morning	Carbs	Lunch	Carbs	Supper	Carbs	Snacks	Carbs

Medications taken today:

Today I am 37 Weeks and 6 Days Pregnant

Date: ______________________________ Day of Week: Su M T W Th F Sa

Morning Weight: ______________________

Exercise: ______________________

Baby Movements or Activity:

____

Today I am

____

Because ______________________________

____

Blood Sugar Tracking:

AM/Fasting: ________ After Lunch: ________

After Breakfast: ________ After Supper: ________

Cesarean Awareness

The rate of cesarean births in the US is high – one in three women give birth surgically. Since cesarean surgery is inherently risky, aiming for a vaginal birth is always better. There are situations, however, when a cesarean may be needed, including maternal illness (pregnancy-induced hypertension, gestational diabetes, or chronic heart or kidney problems), a baby who is positioned head-up or sideways in the uterus, umbilical cord prolapse, placental abruption, placenta previa, non-reassuring fetal heart rate during labor, and cephalopelvic disproportion (baby's head is too big for mom's pelvis). Preparing ahead for complications is the best strategy. Learn more about what cesarean birth is like, and how to make the most of your postpartum recovery and shift to motherhood.

Morning	Carbs	Lunch	Carbs	Supper	Carbs	Snacks	Carbs

Medications taken today:

Today I am 37 Weeks and 7 Days Pregnant

Date: ______________________________ Day of Week: Su M T W Th F Sa

Morning Weight: __________________

Exercise: ____________________

Baby Movements or Activity:

____

Today I am

____

Because ______________________________

____

Blood Sugar Tracking:

AM/Fasting: ________ After Lunch: ________

After Breakfast: ________ After Supper: ________

Pregnancy Traditions: "Slippery" Foods for an Easy Birth

Cultures all over the world have traditions to prepare moms for labor. While some cultures use movement, dance and rituals, others have food recommendations to make the baby's trip through the birth canal simpler. In the Philippines, Tagalog women are instructed to eat many eggs during pregnancy to help the baby slip out. Cherokee mothers in North America traditionally took a bath in water infused with slippery bark, while Mexican women wore snail shell amulets so the baby slipped out as easily as a snail's body slides from the shell. Yemeni midwives feed women oil and milk to ease baby's passage.

Morning	Carbs	Lunch	Carbs	Supper	Carbs	Snacks	Carbs

Medications taken today:

Overview Of My 37th Week:

Doctor's Visits Notes:

A Picture To Remember This Week

Today I am 38 Weeks and 1 Day Pregnant

Date: ______________________________ Day of Week: Su M T W Th F Sa

Morning Weight: __________________

Exercise: ________________________

Baby Movements or Activity:

____

Today I am

____

Because __________________________

____

Blood Sugar Tracking:

AM/Fasting: ________ After Lunch: ________

After Breakfast: ________ After Supper: ________

Nutrition Nugget: Food Safety

When preparing foods, you not only want to choose healthy ingredients, but you want to practice food safety, too. Be sure to wash your hands frequently during food preparation, wash all fruits and vegetables, and avoid cross-contamination between meats and other foods. Refrigerate foods promptly, and discard leftovers after two days. Cook and reheat foods to the proper temperature (above 140°F for cooking and at least 165° F for reheating) to avoid ingesting germs that could harm you and your developing fetus. Avoid consuming unpasteurized juices or milk products; raw sprouts; soft cheeses; raw or undercooked meats, poultry, eggs, fish, or shellfish; and, shark, swordfish, king mackerel, or tilefish.

Morning	Carbs	Lunch	Carbs	Supper	Carbs	Snacks	Carbs

Medications taken today:

Today I am 38 Weeks and 2 Days Pregnant

Date: ______________________________ Day of Week: Su M T W Th F Sa

Morning Weight: ________________

Exercise: ______________________

Baby Movements or Activity:

____

Today I am

____

Because ________________________

____

Blood Sugar Tracking:

AM/Fasting: ________ After Lunch: ________

After Breakfast: ________ After Supper: ________

Pelvic and Abdominal Pain

You feel a sudden sharp pain in your low abdomen, and wonder if something is wrong with your baby. Or maybe you feel like your pelvis is splitting in two, or you feel shooting pain in your groin at random times. All of the changes stem from the growing baby's weight on your bodily structures, and from the release of the hormone, relaxin, which is loosening ligaments to help your body open for birth. These pains are usually sharpest with quick movements, so slow down a little if you are having them regularly. Daily exercise and stretching may help. Pubic bone pain may be more difficult to treat, though warm heat may help, as may a supportive maternity belt. Once your baby is born, these pains should resolve.

Morning	Carbs	Lunch	Carbs	Supper	Carbs	Snacks	Carbs

Medications taken today:

Today I am 38 Weeks and 3 Days Pregnant

Date: ______________________________ Day of Week: Su M T W Th F Sa

Morning Weight: ____________________

Exercise: __________________________

Baby Movements or Activity:

____

Today I am

____

Because ____________________________

____

Oh Baby!

Even though your due date is still two weeks away, your baby could be born at any time. Finally your baby's growth has slowed a little – he's likely close to his birth weight. The average newborn weighs around 7 pounds, and measures about 20 inches from head to toes. Interestingly, your baby's intestines are filled with meconium, a greenish-black, tarry substance that will make up your baby's first bowel movement. Meconium is composed of dead cells, amniotic fluid, and waste products from your baby's liver, pancreas, and gallbladder.

Blood Sugar Tracking:

AM/Fasting: _________ After Lunch: __________

After Breakfast: __________ After Supper: __________

Morning	Carbs	Lunch	Carbs	Supper	Carbs	Snacks	Carbs

Medications taken today:

Today I am 38 Weeks and 4 Days Pregnant

Date: ______________________ Day of Week: Su M T W Th F Sa

Morning Weight: ______________________

Exercise: ______________________

Baby Movements or Activity:

____

Today I am

____

Because ______________________

____

Blood Sugar Tracking:

AM/Fasting: ________ After Lunch: ________

After Breakfast: ________ After Supper: ________

Nutrition Nugget: Eating and Drinking in Labor

Some healthcare facilities limit what women can consume during labor. But since it's such hard work, it's important that a woman in childbirth remains hydrated and energized. Most women naturally eat lightly during early labor, and eventually aren't hungry anymore as labor gets more intense. Before your labor starts, learn more about the policies at your facility. Some hospitals only allow ice chips, while others permit clear fluids throughout labor. The best bet is to stay home as long as you can in labor, and to eat a light meal before you go to your birth location. Try to eat something that packs a huge nutritious punch, but is easy to digest, such as an egg with a piece of whole-grain toast.

Morning	Carbs	Lunch	Carbs	Supper	Carbs	Snacks	Carbs

Medications taken today:

Today I am 38 Weeks and 5 Days Pregnant

Date: ______________________________ Day of Week: Su M T W Th F Sa

Morning Weight: ____________________

Exercise: ____________________

Baby Movements or Activity:

____

Today I am

____

Because ______________________________

____

Blood Sugar Tracking:

AM/Fasting: ________ After Lunch: ________

After Breakfast: ________ After Supper: ________

Breastfeeding Basics

What do you need to know to get breastfeeding off to the best start? Limit pain medications for birth, which can make your baby sleepy for many hours. Pay close attention to positioning and latch – keep baby tightly tummy-to-mummy and wait for a wide-open mouth for latching. Listen for swallows – a sure sign of milk transfer. Expect your milk to come in two to five days after birth, and know that in the meantime, colostrum is just enough for your baby as long as he or she is getting to the breast often. Newborns typically nurse eight to twelve times per 24 hours, and those feedings aren't always evenly spaced. If breastfeeding hurts, or if you're not sure your baby is getting enough, get help from a knowledgeable lactation professional.

Morning	Carbs	Lunch	Carbs	Supper	Carbs	Snacks	Carbs

Medications taken today:

Today I am 38 Weeks and 6 Days Pregnant

Date: ______________________________ Day of Week: Su M T W Th F Sa

Morning Weight: ________________

Exercise: ______________________

Baby Movements or Activity:

____

Today I am

____

Because ___________________________

____

Blood Sugar Tracking:

AM/Fasting: ________ After Lunch: ________

After Breakfast: ________ After Supper: ________

Describe a Contraction

Ask ten women to describe a contraction, and you will get ten very different stories. Contractions are a tightening of the uterus under the influence of the hormone, oxytocin. This spasm pulls up on the uterus, thinning and opening the cervix, and eventually pushes down on baby's body. With each contraction, nerves in the pelvis are stimulated, and ligaments are stretched. All of these changes together provide women with a variety of sensations that can be described in many ways. Rather than focusing on the contraction as painful, transforming it into something beneficial can help women get through. Even just thinking of the contraction in other terms might help. For example, one mother described her contractions as standing in the ocean and allowing waves to crash rhythmically over her then pull back out to sea.

Morning	Carbs	Lunch	Carbs	Supper	Carbs	Snacks	Carbs

Medications taken today:

Today I am 38 Weeks and 7 Days Pregnant

Date: ______________________________ Day of Week: Su M T W Th F Sa

Morning Weight: __________________

Exercise: __________________

Baby Movements or Activity:

____

Today I am

____

Because ______________________________

____

Why Wait?

You're nearing the end of your pregnancy, and your healthcare provider has said your baby is full-term. He's even proposed scheduling an induction– should you take him up on his offer? Unless there is a strong medical reason for induction, it's always best to wait until your baby is ready to be born. Starting labor artificially can lead to stronger contractions, more pain medication use, a greater risk of fetal distress, and a greater likelihood of cesarean birth. If you have a condition such as gestational diabetes or pregnancy-induced hypertension, however, it may be safer for your baby to be born sooner rather than later. Prepare yourself by knowing what to expect with induction, waiting until labor is well underway to use pain medication, and staying as mobile as possible during labor.

Blood Sugar Tracking:

AM/Fasting: ________ After Lunch: ________

After Breakfast: ________ After Supper: ________

Morning	Carbs	Lunch	Carbs	Supper	Carbs	Snacks	Carbs

Medications taken today:

Overview Of My 38th Week:

Doctor's Visits Notes:

A Picture To Remember This Week

Today I am 39 Weeks and 1 Day Pregnant

Date: ______________________________ Day of Week: Su M T W Th F Sa

Morning Weight: ____________________

Exercise: ________________________

Baby Movements or Activity:

____

Today I am

____

Because ______________________________

____

Nutrition Nugget: Herbal Teas

Some herbal teas have benefits specific to pregnant moms. For instance, chamomile tea aids digestion, and dandelion can help with swelling and soothe an upset stomach. Many women with morning sickness rely on ginger root, which can help with nasal congestion, as well. Nettle leaf tea is rich in iron, calcium and other vitamins and minerals. Peppermint tea relieves gas pains and calms the stomach. While most herbs in tea are safe during pregnancy, read labels so you know what's in your cup, and look up herbs or ingredients you are unfamiliar with. You might even look for teas created especially for pregnant moms. Remember to talk to your doctor with any questions.

Blood Sugar Tracking:

AM/Fasting: _________ After Lunch: _________

After Breakfast: _________ After Supper: _________

Morning	Carbs	Lunch	Carbs	Supper	Carbs	Snacks	Carbs

<u>Medications taken today:</u>

Today I am 39 Weeks and 2 Days Pregnant

Date: ______________________________ Day of Week: Su M T W Th F Sa

Morning Weight: __________________

Exercise: _______________________

Baby Movements or Activity:

____

Today I am

____

Because _________________________

____

Blood Sugar Tracking:

AM/Fasting: ________ After Lunch: ________

After Breakfast: ________After Supper: ________

What Is Perineal Massage?

Perineal massage is a way of preparing your tissues for the birth of your baby. Your perineum is the area from the vagina to the anus that the baby needs to pass over during birth. If those tissues are more elastic, you have a greater likelihood of delivering without an episiotomy or tear. Starting this week, massage the area around your vagina each day. Use a natural oil for lubrication, and enough pressure that you can feel a stretching or stinging. Another bonus? This conditions you for the stretching you will feel when your baby's head crowns. You can even include your partner, and make the massage a fun and intimate time.

Morning	Carbs	Lunch	Carbs	Supper	Carbs	Snacks	Carbs

<u>Medications taken today:</u>

Today I am 39 Weeks and 3 Days Pregnant

Date: ______________________________ Day of Week: Su M T W Th F Sa

Morning Weight: ____________________

Exercise: ________________________

Baby Movements or Activity:

____

Today I am

____

Because ___________________________

____

Blood Sugar Tracking:

AM/Fasting: ________ After Lunch: ________

After Breakfast: ________ After Supper: ________

Oh Baby!

The placenta, which has supported all of your baby's needs throughout pregnancy, starts its decline around this time, though it's still strong enough to sustain your baby until birth. His body is starting to produce its own hormones, which will aid the birth process and early bonding. He is still building up fat layers, and putting on weight. Your baby is weighing in at seven to eight pounds, though boys tend to be heavier than girls. Even though he's not putting on much weight, his brain continues to develop.

Morning	Carbs	Lunch	Carbs	Supper	Carbs	Snacks	Carbs

<u>Medications taken today:</u>

Today I am 39 Weeks and 4 Days Pregnant

Date: ______________________________ Day of Week: Su M T W Th F Sa

Morning Weight: __________________

Exercise: _______________________

Baby Movements or Activity:

____

Today I am

____

Because _____________________________

____

Blood Sugar Tracking:

AM/Fasting: ________ After Lunch: ________

After Breakfast: ________ After Supper: ________

Managing Back Labor

Pain in the lower back with and between contractions is often referred to as back labor. Most of the time it is cause by a fetus who is facing mom's front rather than her back so that baby's head puts added pressure on mom's back. Hands and knees positions, walking up stairs and doing lunges may help baby to rotate. If baby is engaged in the pelvis, try the knee-chest position: on your hands and knees, lower your shoulders so your head and arms rest on the bed or floor, allowing gravity to pull baby out of the pelvis just enough to rotate. If baby doesn't turn before birth, he can safely be born "sunny side up," though it will be more painful for mom.

Morning	Carbs	Lunch	Carbs	Supper	Carbs	Snacks	Carbs

Medications taken today:

Today I am 39 Weeks and 5 Days Pregnant

Date: ______________________________ Day of Week: Su M T W Th F Sa

Morning Weight: __________________

Exercise: __________________

Baby Movements or Activity:

____

Today I am

____

Because __________________________

____

Blood Sugar Tracking:

AM/Fasting: ________ After Lunch: _________

After Breakfast: _________After Supper: _________

Breech Baby Basics

While most babies have assumed a head-down position by this time in pregnancy, around four percent of babies never get to that point and are in a breech position (with their bottom or feet closest to the cervix) when labor starts. If your baby is breech at 34 or 35 weeks, there's still a chance he or she can be persuaded into a more favorable position. Try using light or a cold object high on the abdomen – your baby will try to wiggle away from the annoying stimulus. Try playing music near your pubic bone. Consider the breech tilt, where you position yourself with your pelvis higher than your head. Acupuncture, The Webster Technique, and External Cephalic Version are other techniques for turning baby that need to be done by a trained professional.

Morning	Carbs	Lunch	Carbs	Supper	Carbs	Snacks	Carbs

Medications taken today:

Today I am 39 Weeks and 6 Days Pregnant

Date: ______________________ Day of Week: Su M T W Th F Sa

Morning Weight: ______________

Exercise: ______________

Baby Movements or Activity:

____

Today I am

____

Because ______________________

____

Blood Sugar Tracking:

AM/Fasting: ________ After Lunch: ________

After Breakfast: ________ After Supper: ________

Relaxation Quickie - Visualization

Visualization can be a powerful tool in transforming thoughts and sensations. They might be a full script with a story that your partner walks you through during labor, or they might be short mental exercises you use to distract yourself during or between contractions. Try imagining your favorite place and see how many details you can call to mind. Remember with all of your senses, then actively recreate that space mentally during labor. Or more simply, try adding color to your breathing – perhaps inhaling one color and exhaling another, more relaxing or peaceful color. Focusing your thoughts on external stimuli will help you overcome internal stimuli that may be painful or uncomfortable.

Morning	Carbs	Lunch	Carbs	Supper	Carbs	Snacks	Carbs

Medications taken today:

Today I am 39 Weeks and 7 Days Pregnant

Date: ______________________________ Day of Week: Su M T W Th F Sa

Morning Weight: __________________

Exercise: ______________________

Baby Movements or Activity:

____

Today I am

____

Because ___________________________

____

Blood Sugar Tracking:

AM/Fasting: ________ After Lunch: _________

After Breakfast: _________After Supper: _________

What If My Water Breaks?

Some women experience a gush or trickle amniotic fluid as their first sign of labor. Though this only happens in around 10 percent of pregnancies, it is usually followed by contractions. If your water breaks, take note of the time, amount, color, and odor, and call your healthcare provider. If contractions don't start on their own within 18 to 24 hours, your provider may want to use medical means to get labor going. If your amniotic fluid is greenish or brownish, this may indicate your baby has had their first bowel movement insidc, which can lead to respiratory problems in some newborns. If your water doesn't break at the onset of labor, it will usually break on its own at some point before birth.

Morning	Carbs	Lunch	Carbs	Supper	Carbs	Snacks	Carbs

<u>Medications taken today:</u>

Overview Of My 39th Week:

Doctor's Visits Notes:

A Picture To Remember This Week

Today I am 40 Weeks and 1 Day Pregnant

Date: ______________________________ Day of Week: Su M T W Th F Sa

Morning Weight: __________________

Exercise: ____________________

Baby Movements or Activity:

____

Today I am

____

Because ____________________________

____

Blood Sugar Tracking:

AM/Fasting: _________ After Lunch: _________

After Breakfast: _________ After Supper: _________

Water Birth

Have you considered birthing in a tub? Water birth is a safe option with numerous benefits. Water provides all-over support for a laboring woman's body, allowing her to relax all of her muscles. This relaxation can improve blood flow and keep labor progressing evenly. The relaxation afforded by warm water can even help her feel more in control of her labor. Pushing in water may reduce the risk of vaginal tearing. Even just showering or sitting in a warm bath is helpful in relaxing muscles and alleviating pain. So if you don't have access to water birth, at least try to incorporate one of these into your labor.

Morning	Carbs	Lunch	Carbs	Supper	Carbs	Snacks	Carbs

Medications taken today:

Today I am 40 Weeks and 2 Days Pregnant

Date: ______________________________ Day of Week: Su M T W Th F Sa

Morning Weight: __________________

Exercise: __________________

Baby Movements or Activity:

____

Today I am

____

Because _____________________________

____

Blood Sugar Tracking:

AM/Fasting: ________ After Lunch: __________

After Breakfast: __________After Supper: __________

Pelvic Exams in Late Pregnancy

You've been seeing your healthcare provider monthly since the beginning of pregnancy, but starting in the third trimester your visits will be more frequent. Around now, you're likely seeing your doctor or midwife every week, and he or she may be doing internal exams to assess your cervix. Signs he or she is looking for include: ripening or softening of the cervix; dilation (opening of the cervix); effacement (thinning of the cervix); and a change of cervical position (from back to front). Your provider will also assess your baby's location – either high up in the uterus, or engaged and moving down in the pelvis. If your doctor tells you you're 1 cm dilated and 50 percent effaced, don't get too excited yet. You still need regular contractions to finish the process!

Morning	Carbs	Lunch	Carbs	Supper	Carbs	Snacks	Carbs

Medications taken today:

Today I am 40 Weeks and 3 Days Pregnant

Date: ______________________________ Day of Week: Su M T W Th F Sa

Morning Weight: ________________

Exercise: ________________

Baby Movements or Activity:

____

Today I am

____

Because ______________________________

____

Oh Baby!

Finally your due date! Very few babies are actually born on the exact day, though the majority are born within two weeks before or after. Your baby might weigh anywhere from six to nine pounds and be between 19 and 22 inches long. (You might compare him to a small pumpkin.) Fifteen percent of your baby's body weight is now from fat. Experts still don't know exactly what causes labor to start, but when that signal comes, all baby's systems are ready for the outside world. Your little one's skull bones are not yet fused, allowing for some overlap as he moves through the birth canal. This "molding" may cause your baby to look cone-headed for several days after birth.

Blood Sugar Tracking:

AM/Fasting: ________ After Lunch: ________

After Breakfast: ________ After Supper: ________

Morning	Carbs	Lunch	Carbs	Supper	Carbs	Snacks	Carbs

Medications taken today:

Today I am 40 Weeks and 4 Days Pregnant

Date: ______________________________ Day of Week: Su M T W Th F Sa

Morning Weight: __________________

Exercise: ______________________

Baby Movements or Activity:

____

Today I am

____

Because ___________________________

____

Blood Sugar Tracking:

AM/Fasting: ________ After Lunch: _________

After Breakfast: _________After Supper: _________

Movement for Labor

Lying flat on your back throughout labor is the most painful position you can assume. Use gravity to your advantage – let it help move baby down through the pelvis – by staying upright for as much of labor as you can. Try walking, slow dancing, or squatting. If you are tired, semi-reclining positions are better than lying down, and side-lying is better than on your back. If you are feeling pain, try changing positions. Most of the time a simple shift in how you are position goes a long way in relieving pain. No single position will work throughout labor for comfort, so have a variety in mind to try.

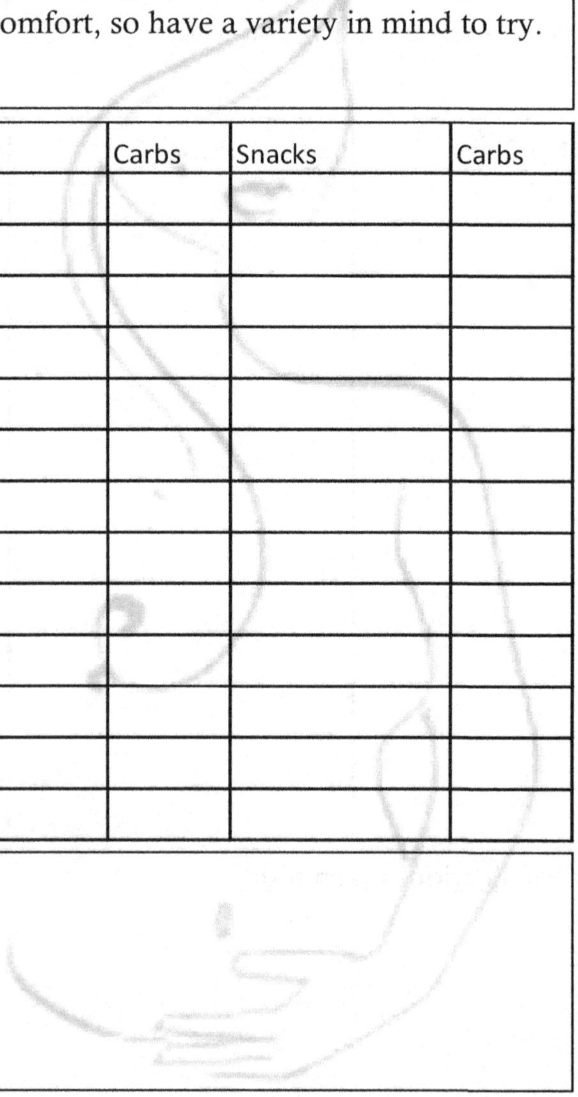

Morning	Carbs	Lunch	Carbs	Supper	Carbs	Snacks	Carbs

Medications taken today:

Today I am 40 Weeks and 5 Days Pregnant

Date: ______________________________ Day of Week: Su M T W Th F Sa

Morning Weight: __________________

Exercise: _______________________

Baby Movements or Activity:

____

Today I am

____

Because ___________________________

____

Blood Sugar Tracking:

AM/Fasting: _________ After Lunch: _________

After Breakfast: _________ After Supper: _________

Keep Mom and Baby Together After Birth

Plan to keep your baby with you as much as possible after birth. The best transition to the outside world is for your baby to remain skin-to-skin with you immediately following delivery. Most hospital routines can be completed with the baby on mom's body. This skin-to-skin time keeps baby warm, regulates oxygenation and heart rate, and even facilitates breastfeeding. Find out if your hospital has rooming-in – keeping your baby with you as much as you can during your hospital stay will help you learn your baby's hunger cues and will even aid you in getting more rest as you recover from birth.

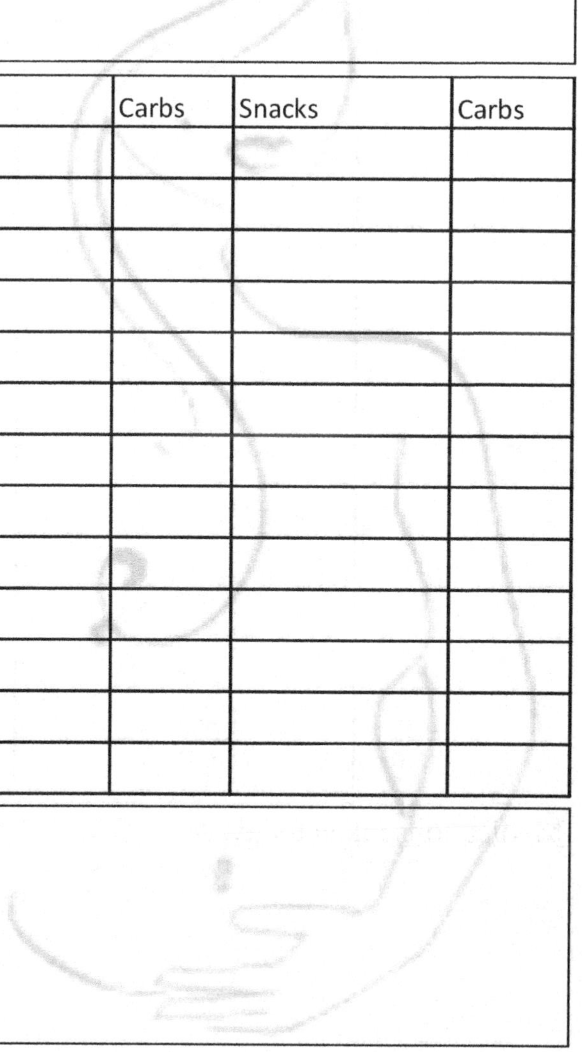

Morning	Carbs	Lunch	Carbs	Supper	Carbs	Snacks	Carbs

Medications taken today:

Today I am 40 Weeks and 6 Days Pregnant

Date: ______________________________ Day of Week: Su M T W Th F Sa

Morning Weight: __________________

Exercise: __________________

Baby Movements or Activity:

____

Today I am

____

Because ____________________________

____

Blood Sugar Tracking:

AM/Fasting: ______ After Lunch: ______

After Breakfast: ______ After Supper: ______

Nutrition Nugget: What to Expect After Birth

Continuing to eat a healthy, well-balanced diet after the birth of your baby is essential for feeling your best. If you're breastfeeding, you will still need some extra calories everyday, so this isn't the time for a crash diet. Eating six small meals each day remains the best strategy for maintaining your energy and managing your blood sugar. Keep nutritious foods on hand that take minimal preparation, and can be eaten with one hand while holding baby in the other. Be sure you are staying hydrated – if you're nursing you may find you are thirsty all the time. One way to be sure you don't skip meals is to spend the last few weeks of pregnancy preparing extra portions that can be frozen until needed postpartum. Then you can just defrost, reheat and enjoy!

Morning	Carbs	Lunch	Carbs	Supper	Carbs	Snacks	Carbs

Medications taken today:

Today I am 40 Weeks and 7 Days Pregnant

Date: ______________________________ Day of Week: Su M T W Th F Sa

Morning Weight: ___________________

Exercise: _______________________

Baby Movements or Activity:

____

Today I am

____

Because ____________________________

____

Blood Sugar Tracking:

AM/Fasting: _________ After Lunch: __________

After Breakfast: _________ After Supper: __________

I'm Past My Due Date!

Ok, so you are past your due date, and you're anxious for your baby to be born. Aside from having your doctor induce your labor, what can you do to get things moving? Several tricks may be worth a try. Nipple stimulation releases oxytocin, as does orgasm, so maybe a little intimacy will bring on some contractions. Semen is also full of prostaglandins, which may help soften the cervix. Castor oil is a folk remedy that has been used for many years when women are past their due date – the thought is that as your bowels are stimulated, your uterus is irritated. Ask your doctor before trying any of these methods to be sure there's no reason for you to wait.

Morning	Carbs	Lunch	Carbs	Supper	Carbs	Snacks	Carbs

Medications taken today:

Overview Of My 40th Week:

Doctor's Visits Notes:

A Picture To Remember This Week

Congratulations!

You made it!

Please send any suggestions for changes to me:

contact@healthydietmenusforyou.com

Made in the USA
Monee, IL
08 November 2026

67388649R10083